MW01632706

The
END
of
CANCER

BY

Charlotte Du Bois
And
John Lubecki

This book has been written to provide up-to-date information related to the material covered and suggestions of ways in which the reader can improve and maintain optimum health. However, anyone using the information and techniques described in this book without the supervision of his doctor does so at his own risk and cannot hold the authors responsible.

This book is sold with the understanding that neither the authors nor the publisher is offering medical advice or any other type of professional services in this publication. Self-treatment can be hazardous; therefore, it is wise to seek out the best available professional help, especially if a serious situation should arise.

© *Charlotte Dubois and John Lubecki 1995*

Published by:
ProMotion Publishing
3368 F Governor Drive
Suite 144
San Diego, CA 92122

(800) 231-1776

All rights reserved. No part of this book may be reproduced in any form or by any means without permission in writing from the publisher.
Library of Congress Catalog Card Number: 88-81875

ISBN1-884030-00-9
Printed in the United States of America.

This book is

dedicated

to the

eradication

of the

scourge of cancer

Introduction

The authors would like it to be clearly understood that they are not involved in any kind of cancer research and do not offer any advice on how cancer should be treated. They are *only reporting* on new discoveries which have been made in holistic medicine and on the way cancer is being successfully treated in European holistic health clinics.

The opinions expressed in this book are not those of the authors. This book is an attempt to synthesize from the available information that which appears to be most relevant and valid.

In this country all harmless unorthodox treatments for cancer are outlawed, leaving only surgery, radiation, or chemotherapy to choose from. It is the opinion of many leading European cancer authorities, who use natural therapies for treating cancer, that orthodox treatments often do far more harm than the cancer itself. They may exhaust the patient's body to such a degree that recovery is no longer possible.

All statements made in this book with regard to the causes of cancer, and to the effective nutritional and other natural methods of treatment of cancer, are well documented—as can be seen from the references. The purpose of this book is to provide a synopsis of the available information, thereby cutting this mass of data down to size and making it more easily accessible to the layman.

It has been said that, "A solution to every conceivable problem has already been found by someone, somewhere. The reason we don't know about it is because of lack of communication." This book is an attempt to help cancer patients, as well as those who want to prevent this dreaded disease, find the information they are seeking more easily—instead of having to wade through an endless mass of literature on the subject.

Most of the material presented has been taken from the books whose names are listed at the end of this introduction. Unless otherwise indicated, the information in this text is derived from these books. The reader is strongly urged to read them. Lack of space makes it impossible to cover all aspects of cancer as fully as necessary. To make this work concise and easy to read, the authors have attempted to explain only the most important features of the holistic treatments available. These books provide more detailed information on most of the topics mentioned.

The majority of the books named can be found in your local lending library or health food store.

BOOKS

*Candida, Silver (Mercury) Fillings and
the Immune System*
by Betsy Russell-Manning, Greensward Press
1600 Larkin #104, San Francisco, CA 94109

World Without Cancer
by G. Edward Griffin, American Media
P.O. Box 4646, Westlake Village, CA 91359

An End To Cancer?
by Leon Chaitow, Thorsons Publishers Limited
Wellingborough, Northhamptonshire, England

The Death of Cancer
by Dr. Harold W. Manner, Advanced Century Publishing
Corporation
P.O. Box 1052 Evanston, IL 60204

A Cancer Therapy, Results of Fifty Cases
by Max Gerson, M.D., Totality Books
P.O. Box 1035, Del Mar, CA 92014

The Cancer prevention Diet
by Michio Kushi, Saint Martins Press
175 5th Ave., New York, NY 10010

The Macrobiotic Approach to Cancer
by Michio Kushi and the East West Foundation
Avery Publishing Group, Inc., Wayne, NJ

The Conquest Of Cancer
by Dr. Virginia Livingston-Wheeler and Edmond G. Addeo,
Franklin Watts,
387 Park Ave. South, New York, NY 10016

The Cancer Answer . . .Nutrition
by Maureen Salaman, Stanford Publishing
1259 El Camino Real, Menlo Park, CA 94025

Cancer and Vitamin C
by Ewan Cameron and Linus Pauling,
The Linus Pauling Institute of Science and Medicine
2700 San Hill Road, Menlo Park, CA 94025

A Challenging Second Opinion
by John A. McDougall, M.D., New Century Publishers, Inc.,
220 Old New Brunswick Road, Piscatoway, NJ 08854

Cancer And Its Nutritional Therapies
by Dr. Richard A. Passwater, Keat's Publishing, Inc.,
27 Pine Street, New Canaan, CT 06840

Cancer: A Healing Crisis
by Jack Tropp, Cancer Book House, Cancer Control Society
2034 N. Berendo, Los Angeles, CA 90027

The Causes And Prevention Of Cancer
by Dr. Frederick B. Levenson, Stein and Day,
Scarborougdh House, Briar Cliff Manor, NY 10510

The Cancer Blackout
by Maurice Natenrbergh, Cancer Control Society,
2043 N. Berendo, Los Angeles, CA 90027

Dr. Kelley's Answer to Cancer
by William D. Kelly, Wedgestone Press
P.O. Box 175, Winfield, KS 671565

How You Can Beat The Killer Diseases
by Harold Harper, M.D., and Michael Culbert
Arlington House Publishers, New Rochelle, NY

Naked Empress—Or The Great Medical Fraud
by Hans Ruesch, Civis-Schweiz Postfach,
323 CH-8030 Zurich, Switzerland

The Great Medical Monopoly Wars
by P. J. Lisa, International Institute
of Natural Health Sciences, Inc.,
P.O. Box 5550, Huntington Beach, CA 92615

Confession Of A Medical Heretic
by Robert S. Mendelsohn, M.D., Warner Books, Inc.,
666 Fifth Ave., New York, NY 10103

The Yeast Connection
by William G. Crook, M.D., Professional Books,
P.O. Box 3494, Jackson, TN 38301

The Yeast Syndrome
by John Parks Trowbridge, M.D., and Morton Walker,
D.P.M., Bantam Books, Inc.,
666 Fifth Ave., New York, NY 10103

The Grape Cure
by Johanna Brandt, Ehret Literature Publishing Co., Inc.,
Dobbs Ferry, NY 10522-0024

Mercury Poisoning From Dental Amalgam—A Hazard To The Human Brain
by Patrick Stortebecker, M.D., Ph.D., Bio-Probe, Inc.,
P.O. Box 58010, Orlando, FL 32858

Dental Caries As A Cause Of Nervous Disorders
by Patrick Stortebecker, M.D., Ph.D., Bio-Probe, Inc.,
P.O. Box 58010, Orlando, FL 32858

Silver Dental Fillings—The Toxic Time Bomb
by San Ziff, Aurora Press,
205 Third Ave. 2A, New York, NY 10003

The Chelation Answer
by Morton Walker, D.P.M., M. Evans and Company, Inc.,
216 East 49th Street, New York, NY 10017

Bypassing Bypass
by Elmer Cranton, M.D., and Arline Brecher, Stein and Day
Scarborough House, Briarcliff Manor, NY 10510

Infertility & Birth Defects
by Sam Ziff and Dr. Michael F. Ziff, Bio-Probe Inc.,
P.O. Box 58010, Orlando, FL 32858

CONTENTS

1   Escape From The Grip Of Modern Medicine

Charlotte's Story

The lump in my breast had reached the size of an egg and had been acutely painful for several months before I finally found the courage to go to a doctor. The growth had first been discovered during a routine medical checkup in the summer of 1985. It was only about two centimeters in diameter at the time but the doctor was very concerned. She insisted that I have a biopsy to determine, as soon as possible, whether we were dealing with a malignancy or a benign condition.

The thought of having medical tests filled me with fear. I had worked in nursing as a medical assistant in a large hospital for twenty years and had seen many cancer patients. It is common knowledge that invasive medical tests may cause cancer to spread. The doctor attempted to calm my fears by suggesting I have a needle aspiration. She explained that this is the safest of all the tests for cancer and cannot possibly do any harm. But I knew this was not true. I remembered several cases where cancer started growing rapidly even following needle aspirations. To the doctor's distress, I refused to listen and declined all the standard tests she suggested, with the exception of a mammogram. This X-ray of my breast proved inconclusive, however. The radiologist said that it was impossible to say whether the tumor was malignant because he could not see part of it clearly enough. In his opinion there was a fifty-fifty chance that the tumor was cancerous.

Apart from this I would not agree to any further tests. I knew, that if they proved positive, the doctors would insist on treatment. The thought of having chemotherapy, radiation or surgery filled me with fear. Unfortunately, these are the only treatments used by orthodox doctors.

I had seen numerous patients undergoing chemotherapy. Many of them were in pitiful condition— weak, glassy-eyed, without hair and without hope. Their pale faces, groans of pain and looks of despair were enough to make a healthy person sick. I had often heard doctors say that chemotherapy rarely succeeds in curing cancer. At best, it might help a patient stay alive a little longer.

The patients who were especially sensitive to the poisonous drugs used in chemotherapy often developed symptoms such as violent vomiting for hours on end, bloody diarrhea, complete hair loss, impaired vision and hearing, extreme weakness, ulceration of the mouth and other parts of the body, sterility and loose teeth.

I remembered one middle-aged patient especially well. He was in such terrible condition, that when his wife saw him, she was horrified and asked, "I wonder which is going to kill my husband first, the cancer or the treatment?" This patient did not come back for more chemotherapy. We later learned that he eventually managed to get well with diets, vitamins, and other natural therapies. When the doctors at the hospital heard this, they said he probably had a spontaneous remission and would have recovered no matter what had been done. They would not admit natural methods could have helped.

Radiation can be as deadly as chemotherapy. It is true that cancer cells cannot survive radiation and are soon destroyed, but radiation can also cause damage to important structures and organs. Worst of all, it has a devastating effect on the patient's immune system which is his chief defense against the cancer.

Surgery seemed to me to be the least dangerous of the orthodox treatments for cancer and gave the best chance of recovery, especially if only a minor operation would do the trick. However, surgery also has its problems. The worst is that it can hasten the growth of the cancer and cause it to spread. Cancer surgery can also disfigure the body unbelievably. I remembered seeing countless unfortunate people with huge scars on their faces and necks, amputated limbs, mastectomies, colostomies and other crippling mutilations. Cancer surgery leaves behind a trail of cripples creeping back from the halls of horror.

If cancer surgery was at least guaranteed to cure the problem forever, the pain and suffering would perhaps be worthwhile, but this is not so. In fact, the very opposite is often true. Surgery exhausts and depresses the patient and weakens him even further. This makes it still more difficult for his body to fight the cancer and frequently nothing is achieved. The cancer merely kills the weakened patient faster. In short, surgery removes only the symptom, the tumor itself, but offers no guarantee of a cure. The underlying problem, the reason the cancer developed in the first place, remains uncorrected.

Worst of all, like everyone else, specialists can make mistakes. They may carve up a perfectly healthy individual because there is a suspicion of cancer and because they are terrified of a malpractice suit. Cases like this probably make up a large proportion of the so called "successes" of modern medicine. The following story is a good example of this. A lady M.D. discovered a lump in her breast. The lump was removed surgically, but before the operation the patient was asked to sign a release saying that she agreed to more radical surgery if the lump was found to be malignant. She refused and told the surgeon she wanted more time to decide what exactly would have to be done if this turned out to be the case. When she awakened following the operation, the surgeon came in and said that the lump had in fact been found to be malignant. He regretted the patient had not agreed to allow him to perform more extensive surgery. Greatly upset at this news, the lady M.D. asked that the lab test for malignancy be repeated. This time the result of the test came back negative. The test was repeated twice more. It was negative both times.

From this it can be seen that biopsy results are not always reliable. Although the slides do show the cells taken from some patients to be definitely malignant, and those from other patients to be clearly normal, there is a considerable grey area in between. The result is that doctors sometimes have to guess what should be done.

When I considered the alternatives, I felt very uneasy. The prospect of being a guinea pig did not appeal to me in the least. Many times I had heard that cancer patients frequently live much longer if they do not have orthodox treatments. Electing to be treated for cancer by conventional doctors can sometimes be equivalent to a sophisticated way of committing suicide.

However, not all patients blindly follow the advice of their doctors and submit like sheep to the barbaric conventional therapies. I knew of a number of people who had escaped from the grip of organized medicine and had been successfully treated in Europe and the Mexican cancer clinics. These people had to travel abroad because they could find no one in this country to help them with their incurable health problems. Among them were individuals suffering with not only cancer but other serious conditions such as rheumatoid arthritis, lupus, multiple sclerosis, and other supposedly incurable ailments. Amazingly, many of these patients came back after a comparatively short time completely cured of their infirmities. From speaking to some of them and their families, I had learned of the wonderful results which were being obtained with the use of diets, cleansing, Laetrile, homeopathic remedies and other natural methods.

What interested me most at the time was a blood test for cancer which was being used by the Mexican clinics. This test was just what I was looking for. It was simple, non-invasive, and most important of all, it could not harm my health. It did not cause the cancer to spread and did not weaken the body. Early in 1986, I went to Mexico and had the first of these blood tests for cancer. To my great relief, it was inconclusive. The doctor said that if I did indeed have cancer, it was inactive at present and it would probably be a long time before it began growing and became life threatening. He advised me to come back in three months to have the test repeated. The lump had not changed in appearance since its discovery six months earlier and I began hoping it was benign and would not cause me further problems.

My health started deteriorating seriously two years before the discovery of the lump in my breast. I developed frequent headaches, depression, fatigue, confusion, memory loss, insomnia, and pains in my chest, legs and back. It became increasingly difficult for me to work, but I could not give up my job at the hospital because of financial problems. By the time the lump was first noticed, the above symptoms were joined by severe digestive problems and an inexplicable feeling of anxiety. I became irritable, short-tempered, unable to relax and felt I was heading for a nervous breakdown.

Now, the hope that perhaps I did not have cancer and the warm spring weather brought about an improvement in my health. It was not until the autumn of that year that things began to take a decisive turn for the worse. Towards the end of October, I became very ill and decided to have another blood test in Mexico. The test was inconclusive as a result of an intestinal infection and the doctor asked me to come back and have it repeated as soon as the infection was under control.

Soon after this second trip to Mexico, I noticed that the lump suddenly began growing rapidly. My breast became inflamed, swollen and painful. However, I did not go back to Mexico until the spring of 1987. This was partly because I was afraid the doctor would tell me that I had cancer and partly because my infection would not clear up. By then the lump had become so large it was easily noticeable under my clothing. This time the test was definitely positive and the doctor said there could be no further doubt that the lump was malignant.

All hope that I did not have cancer now vanished and I was faced with the agonizing decision of what to do next. As far as I was concerned, all orthodox therapies were out. After watching doctors treat thousands of patients, I had made up my mind that there was no way they would do any of these things to me. I did not even remotely consider having surgery, chemotherapy, radiation or any other orthodox treatment. But neither did I have a clear plan of action if the lump in my breast was found to be malignant. Now there was no more time to lose. A decision had to be make quickly or soon it would be too late, if it was not too late already.

For the time being, I spent another week in Mexico as an outpatient at the clinic. When the doctor had finished all the tests, he explained that my cancer was basically due to the following problems which had been developing over the years: (1) the toxic condition of my body, (2) a breakdown of my immune system, (3) mercury poisoning from my amalgam fillings, (4) a severe infestation with intestinal parasites and (5) candida, or a yeast overgrowth.

The doctor said that it is now widely recognized among holistic practitioners that cancer is not a true disease. It is a symptom of extreme toxicity and a depressed immune system. When the body becomes rundown and can no longer cope with the accumulations of poisons in the tissues, tumors begin to grow.

The doctor told me that the extremely toxic condition of my body was mainly the result of the parasitic infestation and the candida. He explained that researchers had now found that mercury poisoning caused by amalgam fillings plays an important part in predisposing people to yeast overgrowth. The mercury from the amalgam fillings spreads to all parts of the body, especially the brain and kidneys, and severely depresses the body's immune system.

The doctor recommended a cleansing program and gave me bee propolis tablets from Germany, Laetrile tablets, herbs, and homeopathic remedies. I was to take these daily and return to the clinic in two months. In the meantime, I was to follow a strict diet of fresh fruits, vegetables and cereals prepared from millet, brown rice, quinoa grains, and corn. I was also allowed occasional servings of fish or turkey, fresh raw butter, fresh herbs and small quantities of cold pressed oils. Strictly forbidden were all red meats, pasteurized milk, chicken, processed foods, fried foods, salt and other seasonings.

The doctor told me to have the highly toxic amalgam fillings removed from my teeth as soon as possible, and replaced with composites and other non-toxic materials. However, he did not know of a dentist in my area where I could go to have this done. Although in Europe and some other countries it is recognized that mercury can cause serious health problems, the dentists in the United States are still not in agreement in this respect. It is therefore, difficult to find a dentist who understands the problem and knows what materials to use in place of the amalgam.

My immediate concern was a shortage of the money needed to cover the expenses of the treatment. I knew that if I could spend a month or two at the clinic in Mexico, I would have a good chance of getting well. However, I could not afford this myself. Neither did my health insurance cover the costs of treatment in the Mexican cancer clinics, or any of the other places where natural therapies are used. It covered only the cost of conventional therapies—surgery, radiation and chemotherapy—all of which I already knew from experience to be short cuts to the grave. Even if it was covered by insurance, the thought of martyrdom at the hands of conventional doctors made me shudder. However, if I was to get well, I would somehow have to find enough money to pay for not only the cancer treatment but also for the dental work. The doctor at the clinic in Mexico had told me that unless the extremely toxic silver fillings were removed from my teeth, I may not recover. He felt that the cleansing program alone might not be sufficient.

The solution to my financial dilemma was provided by my mother. She said she would gladly cover the costs of any therapies I needed to have. I will be eternally grateful to her for this. Without her help, I am certain I would never have made it. My cancer was so advanced by then, that if all the recommendations the doctor made had not been followed, my chances for recovery might have been slim indeed. My mother was my chief supporter, not only financially, but also in helping me to implement the program which eventually led to my recovery.

When I returned home I went back to my job at the hospital, although trying to work in my weakened condition required superhuman willpower. In my free time I started a frantic search for a dentist in my area who would remove the poisonous amalgam from my teeth.

It was not until the second half of April that a friend told me of a holistic medical doctor who had recently come from abroad and started a practice in California. My friend suggested that I contact this doctor as he would be likely to know of a dentist who could do the work I needed. The following morning I called the doctor and was overjoyed when he told me he knew of a very good dentist whose office was about a two-hour drive from my home. He said that this dentist had studied both in Germany and Sweden and was familiar with the dangers presented by mercury fillings. Another advantage was that he used electro-diagnosis, a remarkably accurate diagnostic method developed in Germany. When the doctor heard I had cancer, he suggested that before going to see the dentist I should come to his office and have him check me. He said that he too used electro-diagnosis and had a number of new homeopathic remedies for cancer recently developed in Europe. He made an appointment for me the following day.

When I arrived, the doctor started by checking me with his electronic instrument. This method is considered by many to be the greatest breakthrough ever made in diagnosis. It is far more accurate than the diagnostic methods used by orthodox medicine.

When he had finished his examination, the doctor confirmed that I had cancer. However, he assured me that unless treatment is started too late, cancer is now one of the easier conditions to cure. He said that the nutritional program I had been given by the doctor in Mexico was very good and suggested that I also take two different kinds of homeopathic remedies which would help me recover a lot faster. He said that homeopathic remedies had been used in Europe with good results for many years and doctors familiar with homeopathy had been treating patients with different kinds of cancer with success for a long time.

The doctor told me electro-diagnosis also showed I had intestinal parasites, a yeast overgrowth and mercury poisoning from the amalgam fillings in my teeth. He said cancer patients are commonly found to have candida and parasites. It is believed these organisms play an important part in depressing the body's immune system and causing malignancies. Parasites and candida cause more toxic waste in the body than almost anything else.

I had my first appointment with my new dentist on June 23, 1987. The doctor checked my teeth with his electronic instrument and told me I had five basic problems: (1) the mercury fillings would have to be removed and replaced with non-toxic materials, (2) my gold crowns would have to be redone since some amalgam had been left underneath them, (3) all the teeth with root canals would have to be extracted since they were causing a low grade infection, (4) the amalgam tattoos, areas where the gum tissue had become infiltrated with mercury from the fillings, would have to be cut out, and (5) my porcelain crowns would also have to be replaced since their metal jackets were made of a nickel alloy. Nickel is one of the most carcinogenic materials discovered so far.

The tumor in my breast stopped growing soon after I started the cleansing program. However, it did not begin shrinking immediately. It remained the same size for the next two and a half months. During this time, it was still painful and the soreness caused me considerable discomfort and anxiety. However, when I visited the clinic in Mexico for my follow-up examination , the doctor told me his tests showed the tumor to be no longer active. It had been killed by the Laetrile and the homeopathic remedies.

The first visible change in the size of the tumor occurred when the work on my teeth began. Each time I went to the dentist he would ask me whether the tumor was smaller. He felt that in many cases cancer is caused by mercury from amalgam fillings or other toxic materials, chiefly nickel, placed in teeth by dentists. This, he believed, was one of the reasons for the explosive increase in the number of cancer cases in modern times. He pointed out that at the turn of the century only one person in twenty died of cancer. Now, thanks to modern medicine, it is more like one in four.

It was not until after the removal of some of the larger amalgam fillings that the tumor began to shrink rapidly and stopped causing me discomfort. By the time all the work on my teeth was finished, my tumor had shrunk to only a small lump the size of a pea. The blood tests were negative and electro-diagnosis showed no signs of cancer. My doctors assured me that my cancer was gone and there was no danger of its returning. My general health had also improved tremendously and the symptoms I had been suffering with for over three years stopped. The backaches, stiffness, digestive problems and fatigue were all gone. I felt better than I had in years.

Cancer is the most horrible disease of modern times. Now that I have recovered and this nightmare is behind me, I feel it is my duty to do everything I can to help others. At present, the prospect of dying of cancer haunts most people living in civilized countries. Orthodox medicine offers no hope. On the contrary, it makes matters much worse. The useless treatments used on cancer victims are so horrible, they make the fear of cancer even greater. The family savings are wiped out in a short time, while the stricken patient dies a slow, agonizing death.

But from now on this need not be the case. Therapies developed by holistic doctors in Europe can now be used to cure cancer with amazing ease. In fact, cancer has now become one of the most treatable and preventable diseases. No one need die of cancer any more. It is the purpose of this book to make people aware of the tremendous advances made in holistic medicine, and the hope these new discoveries carry for those countless millions who would otherwise have to succumb to this dreaded disease.

I first became interested in cancer therapies when my best friend Rachel had breast cancer in 1972. Rachel and I had been close friends for a long time. Her illness was a great blow to me. When the results of the biopsy came back, the doctor told us that Rachel had a rare, fast growing, invasive kind of cancer which seldom started in the breast.

After the biopsy Rachel had a hard time regaining consciousness. When she eventually recovered she was wheeled off to her car, but passed out again on her way home. This happened several more times during the next day or two. When her daughter called the hospital, a nurse told her that this was due to Rachel's being overly sensitive to the anesthetic the doctor had given her. The doctor who gave Rachel the anesthesia was the same anesthesiologist who several months later gave a young man in her town an overdose. The young man never regained consciousness. Rachel's time had not arrived yet.

The result of the biopsy was not communicated to Rachel for two weeks. When it was, all arrangements had already been made for her to go into the hospital to have her breast removed. However, when Rachel asked the doctor about the chances of the surgery being successful, he openly told her he thought it would not help. He felt there was no point in removing her breast since the cancer had already spread to other parts of her body. Therefore, one surgery after another would have to be performed and the doctor did not want to cut her up.

When the medical doctor told her he could do nothing for her, Rachel tried to help herself with natural methods. She came across a book entitled "One Answer to Cancer" by Dr. William Kelley, and started following the recommendations outlined as closely as she could. After three months of coffee enemas, juices, raw foods, and cleansing, Rachel went back to the hospital hoping the tests would show her cancer was better. But there was no change in her condition and the doctor told her she was now terminal and nothing further could be done for her.

Upon hearing this, Rachel decided to go to Mexico and try Laetrile. It was her last hope. She went to Dr. Contreras' clinic in Tiajuana and was given Laetrile injections, while on her own she continued the diet recommended in Dr. Kelley's book. Within a month Rachel improved sufficiently to return home. She took with her enough Laetrile, both injections and tablets, to last her three months. Rachel's cancer was totally under control at the end of this period and when she went back to the hospital, the doctor could find no trace of the malignancy.

After reading many books on cancer, especially Dr. Gerson's book, "A Cancer Therapy- Results of Fifty Cases," I became convinced that cancer is mainly caused by the body becoming overloaded with toxins. The discovery that I had cancer myself was, therefore, a great shock to me. Since I had given up all junk foods long ago, and was careful to eat practically nothing but health foods, I was certain I would never get cancer. But I had failed to take mercury fillings, nickel crowns, intestinal parasites and candida into account. These problems are a far more dangerous source of poisons than even the worst junk foods. I feel certain that if I'd had my mercury fillings removed in time and been careful to keep the parasites and candida under control, I would never have developed cancer.

In spite of the tremendous amount of knowledge about cancer which has been accumulated by holistic doctors in Europe, the final victory over this killer may still have been impossible had it not been for the discovery of electro-diagnosis and muscle-testing. It is electro-diagnosis and muscle-testing which have finally made it possible for us to diagnose patients' problems accurately. They have eliminated the guess work and given us a clear understanding of the true causes of disease. In the next chapter, I will attempt to explain electro-diagnosis and muscle-testing in simple, nontechnical terms which the layman can easily understand.

2   Electro-Diagnosis And Muscle-Testing

Electro-diagnosis is an exciting new form of medical diagnosis developed in Germany. This method enables the doctor to detect cancer in its earliest stages, with a degree of accuracy which could not be achieved before. What is even more important, electro-diagnosis also provides an accurate way of determining not only what caused the malignancy, but what should be done to cure it. The doctors who use this new method consider it the greatest breakthrough ever made in medical science. They predict that when electro-diagnosis becomes more widely used, cancer will be eradicated.

The main purpose of this book is to explain how electro-diagnosis works and how it can be used. If a solution to the cancer problem is to be found, it is important that the public learns as much as possible about new developments in the field of diagnosis and prevention of disease.

Although the number of doctors—medical doctors, homeopaths, dentists, chiropractors, and others—who use electro-diagnosis is rapidly increasing, few lay people have ever heard of it and most doctors still know very little or nothing at all about this new procedure. As has often been the case with other important discoveries in the past, electro-diagnosis has met with strong opposition in some quarters. It has not received the coverage it deserves in the press, whether medical or lay, and there have been a number of cases where doctors have had the electronic instruments used in electro-diagnosis confiscated or destroyed by government agents. Even Dr. Voll, the famous German homeopath who was a candidate for the Nobel Prize in medicine in 1984, was taken to court in Germany when he first began using electro-diagnosis to determine what was wrong with patients. It was only after a great deal of expense and trouble that he was allowed to use this new form of diagnosis without further harassment. Organized medicine's attitude in this respect is a most unfortunate example of "condemnation without investigation." Nearly every single discovery meets with such furious opposition from the medical fraternity that it is a miracle medicine has advanced at all.

Much of the early work on electro-diagnosis was done by Dr. Voll. The electronic instrument he uses in his work is called a dermatron. It was the first instrument of its kind ever used for electro-diagnosis. Many similar instruments have been manufactured since then—some of them in the United States. (See illustration at end of chapter.)

Traditional medical diagnostic methods depend mainly on the doctor's experience and his ability to interpret information gained from the use of scientific instruments or lab tests. This is not true of electro-diagnosis. By making it possible to monitor the flow of energy along the meridians, this new method enables the doctor to "tune into the patient's body" and detect its reactions to different stimuli.

For instance, if a remedy (vitamin, mineral, homeopathic remedy, drug, etc.) is helpful, the electronic instrument shows an immediate improvement in the flow of energy in the patient's body. The opposite happens when a substance which is harmful to the patient is tested. The presence of the harmful substance interferes with the flow of energy along the meridians and the imbalance of energy increases.

In other words, all those factors which are helpful in balancing a person's body, improve the readings on the electronic instrument, while those which are harmful, increase the imbalance and make the readings worse.

By using this simple discovery, human error can be eliminated. Since the body never makes mistakes, by using electro-diagnosis the doctor can find out exactly what should be done to normalize the flow of energy along the meridians and balance the patient's body. He no longer has to rely entirely on his own judgement. The reactions of the patient's body to different stimuli tell him exactly what is wrong and what should be done to correct the problem.

To have a clear understanding of how electro-diagnosis is used as a diagnostic tool, one has to have some understanding of the principles of acupuncture and the laws upon which Eastern Medicine is based.

Many thousands of years ago the Chinese had already discovered that energy passes to all parts of the body along invisible pathways, known as meridians, located just under the surface of the skin. The exact course of the twenty-six meridians discovered by the Chinese, and the precise locations of the acupuncture points on the meridians, is shown on ancient Chinese charts. (See illustration at the end of this chapter.) Some of these charts are many thousands of years old.

To detect changes in the flow of energy along the meridians, the Chinese use pulse diagnosis. This way they are able to discover whether the energy in a person's body is balanced or whether some of the meridians are oversupplied with energy. By using this method, the Chinese can detect imbalances of energy as soon as they occur, and long before symptoms have time to manifest.

For over five thousand years it has been known in China that *health problems cannot develop if the energy in the body is evenly distributed and is flowing smoothly along the meridians.* Symptoms such as headaches, fatigue or back pain are indications that there is interference with the energy flow. Many thousands of years ago, the NEI CHING, the classic of ancient Chinese medicine stated, *"A healthy and well-balanced person is not affected by disease."*

Therefore, the main purpose of the treatments used by the Chinese acupuncturists, regardless of the nature of the symptoms, is to bring the flow of energy in the patient's body back to normal. The acupuncturist knows that, if he can accomplish this, the patient will soon improve.

As a result, Chinese medicine is mainly preventative in nature. The Chinese do not wait until they are sick before going to their doctor; they go to him while they are still well. The doctor's duty is to keep his patients in good health by correcting imbalances of energy before damage has been done and symptoms appear. If a patient does happen to develop health problems, this is considered to be the doctor's fault. He failed to discover energy imbalances in the patient's body before symptoms began. The doctor, therefore, has to treat the patient without charge until he is well again. How wonderful it would be if this was the practice in all countries.

It is only recently that acupuncture has begun to be used in Western countries. Unfortunately, it is mainly used for the relief of pain and not for the prevention of health problems, as is the case in China.

The first Western doctors to use acupuncture principles for purposes other than the relief of pain are German medical doctors who use electro-diagnosis and American doctors (mostly dentists and chiropractors) who use muscle-testing as a diagnostic aid. The reason is that, like pulse diagnosis, both electro-diagnosis and muscle-testing provide an accurate means of detecting energy imbalances as soon as they occur.

Since electro-diagnosis has been discovered, the German doctors who use this new method have also found that symptoms soon begin to disappear when the energy flow in a person's body can be brought back to normal. Cancer is no exception to this rule. Unless too much damage has been done, and the body is no longer able to recover, cancer patients improve rapidly once their bodies have been balanced. This is accomplished by removing the different factors which were interfering with normal energy flow along the meridians.

Organized medicine's failure to recognize the value of the different forms of diagnoses and therapy used by the Chinese is perhaps the most important reason why no satisfactory cure for cancer has been found. When Western doctors learn more about the balancing techniques which have proved themselves to be so effective in China, the Far East, and more recently in Europe, cancer will become a disease of the past—and so will the majority of other health problems which have plagued us for so long. For instance, at present medical doctors cannot even prevent some of the most common conditions. Often they have to limit their treatment to dispensing pain killers, tranquilizers, or muscle relaxants *because they do not clearly understand the causes of these problems.* This is not true of Chinese medicine. *When symptoms are looked upon as the result of energy imbalances, it is easy to discover the underlying causes.* The NEI CHING says:

> "The superior physician helps before the early budding of disease. The inferior physician begins to help when the disease has already set in. Since his help comes when disease has already developed it is said of him that he is ignorant."

What the author of the NEI CHING is trying to say in the above passage is that the doctor should be able to correct imbalances of energy in his patient's body before the patient is aware that something is wrong. The inferior physician cannot detect malfunctions until it is too late and symptoms have already appeared.

Unfortunately, many Western doctors know very little or nothing about the energy flow in the body. Consequently, their diagnoses are only partly correct or entirely wrong. In the long run their efforts to help often do more to unbalance the energy and harm the patient's body than they do to help.

As long as organized medicine continues searching for a cure for cancer the way it has in the past, the slightest hope cannot exist that a cure will ever be found. On the other hand, when doctors begin to view cancer *as only a symptom of energy imbalance* and learn how to detect these imbalances, cancer will cease to exist. No one will suffer from this dreaded disease anymore, and if they do it will be detected and cured before symptoms appear. The German doctors who use electro-diagnosis have been curing cancer patients this way for years. They seldom have to see a cancer patient more than a few times.

Electro-diagnosis and muscle-testing have shown that the four main factors which cause interference with the flow of energy in the body are: (1) deficiencies of vitamins and minerals, (2) sensitivities, (3) toxicity and (4) misalignments of the skeleton. In the case of cancer patients the main causes of interference are invariably toxicity and sensitivities. If you can keep your body reasonably well-balanced and free of toxins, the risk of cancer is greatly reduced.

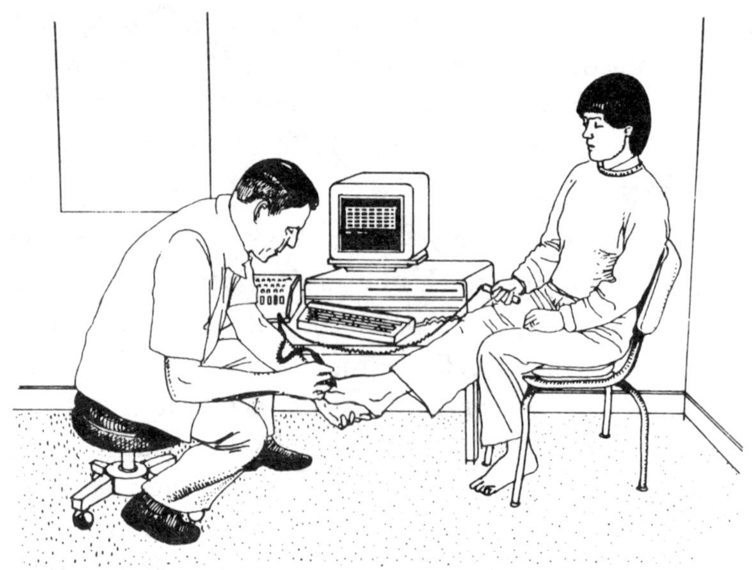

This illustration shows a patient being checked with electro-diagnosis. She is holding one terminal of the electronic instrument—which can be seen in the back—in her hand, while the doctor places the other terminal on an acupuncture point on her foot. The readings on the dial of the instrument tell the doctor how the patient's body is reacting to different stimuli.

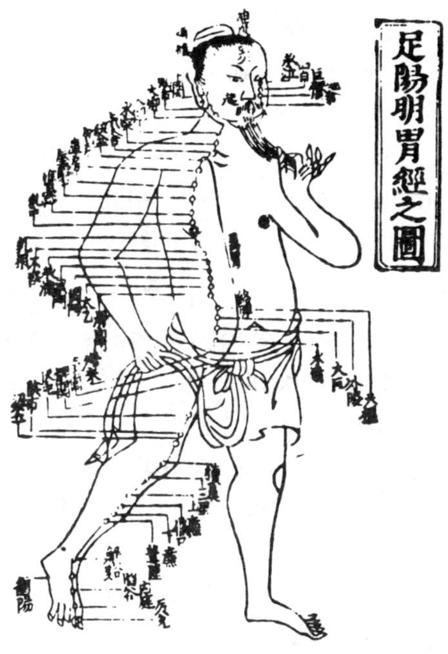

This is a drawing of an ancient Chinese acupuncture chart which shows the points on the stomach meridian. This chart is believed to be over three thousand years old.

The Chinese discovered that there are altogether twenty-six meridians which carry energy to all parts of the body, twelve on each side of the body and two in the center. It is important to understand that the meridian flow is a continuous energy stream. The meridians are interconnected and form a continuous energy pathway. It is amazing that the Chinese had already discovered many thousands of years ago that the energy in the body circulates along these invisible channels.

Muscle-Testing

At the same time that electro-diagnosis was being developed in Europe, a new diagnostic method known as muscle-testing began to be used in the United States. The value of muscle-testing depends on the discovery that, like electro-diagnosis and Chinese pulse diagnosis, it too can be used to detect changes in the meridian energy flow.

Muscle-testing, often referred to as Applied Kinesiology, is a sensational diagnostic procedure developed in recent years. It differs from other methods in that it provides a means of obtaining an immediate response from the body itself. This response tells us with absolute certainty what is wrong and what should be done to correct a health problem.

This means that we no longer have to rely entirely on human expertise and judgement. Instead, we can "ask" the body itself what should be done to help restore it to normal function and good health. Since the body knows exactly what it needs, in many respects muscle-testing is vastly superior to traditional methods of diagnosis.

Muscle-testing has made it possible to discover many important new facts about health. It has shown that the actual causes of health problems are often very different from what we thought in the past.

How Applied Kinesiology Was Developed

Applied Kinesiology is a scientific procedure used for checking the strength of the major muscles of the body. This is done by using specific tests which are designed in such a way that each muscle can be isolated and its strength checked individually. The usual practice is to check the strength of similar muscles on each side of the body. When a noticeable difference in strength is discovered, a muscle on one side of the body being significantly stronger or weaker than the corresponding muscle on the other side, this is interpreted as a sign that something is wrong.

Muscle-testing was originally developed to help patients with problems resulting from the weakness of certain muscles or muscle groups. For instance it was used on patients who had been involved in accidents, individuals with poor posture and on victims of diseases which had resulted in muscle weakness.

Once it had been determined, by using muscle-testing, which muscles needed attention, measures were taken to restore them to normal strength. Physical therapy and special exercises were most frequently recommended to strengthen the weak muscles. As the patient improved, his progress could be monitored by using muscle-testing at regular intervals. This way it could be determined whether or not the weak muscles were responding to treatment.

Originally, muscle-testing did not arouse a great deal of interest. Only a small number of doctors and physical therapists learned about the tests. The usefulness of muscle-testing seemed to be very limited and it was difficult to see how it could be used for any purpose other than a restricted number of conditions.

The Great Discovery

This general lack of interest in muscle-testing would most probably have continued indefinitely, and muscle-testing would never have been more widely used, had it not been for an important discovery. Doctors using this method began noticing that muscle weakness is not just caused by injuries or poor physical condition. They discovered that there are numerous other reasons why muscles may be weak.

Why Muscles Become Weak

When doctors using muscle-testing began checking apparently healthy individuals they were surprised to find that these people also displayed marked differences in muscle strength. At first they could not understand why such large differences in muscle strength occurred in persons who showed no obvious signs of any health problems. But it soon became apparent that differences in muscle strength are mostly due to changes in the energy flow along the acupuncture meridian system. They are not necessarily caused by injuries. If the energy flow decreases, because of interference, the muscles which depend on it become weaker. When it improves, as the factors which interfere with it are corrected, these muscles immediately become stronger (sometimes the increase in strength is as much as 300 to 400 percent.

In his book, "Your Body Does Not Lie," John Diamond, M.D., describes a scientific test in which a Cybex dynamometer was used to record changes in muscle strength on a graph. Amazingly, this instrument recorded reductions to about half strength when weakening stimuli (such as eating refined sugar, thinking unpleasant thoughts or listening to popular rock-and-roll music) were introduced.

From the above it can be seen that the changes in muscle strength, which result from fluctuations in the rate of energy flow along the meridian system, are large enough to be easily detectable. Consequently, like Chinese pulse-diagnosis, muscle-testing can be used as a reliable diagnostic tool for detecting the causes of interference with the meridian energy flow.

Muscle-testing is now used widely by chiropractors, dentists, nutritionists and even some medical doctors. It has proved itself to be a very reliable tool for detecting causes of interference with the meridian energy flow. Thanks to the discovery of the usefulness of muscle-testing, great numbers of patients, who could not be helped before, recovered when the causes of their problems were finally correctly diagnosed.

SUMMARY

This is by far the most important chapter in the book. If you understand the ideas explained clearly, you need have no fear of getting cancer. It is well worth repeating the most important of these principles.

1. It is impossible to be sick if your body is balanced and the flow of energy along the meridians is normal.
2. All sickness is the result of interference with the energy flow along the meridians. If this interference can be corrected, the patient will always get well, unless treatment is started too late.
3. Cancer is nothing but a symptom of energy imbalance. If you keep your body balanced you cannot have cancer.

Fortunately, the number of doctors in Western countries who use electro-diagnosis and muscle-testing is increasing rapidly. Finding such a doctor should soon be within the reach of anyone interested in these new methods.

3   The Causes And Treatment Of Cancer

As we saw in the last chapter, the basic, underlying cause of cancer is an imbalance of energy in the body. If an imbalance is not present for a long time cancer cannot develop, with the exception of some skin cancers which are entirely localized forms of cancer. The imbalance of energy cannot, however, cause cancer by itself. First, the body's immune system has to break down and secondly, the area where the tumor develops has to be subjected to prolonged irritation—often over many years.

It has been known for a long time that the body's immune system plays an important part in protecting us from cancer, in a similar way to that in which it helps protect us from other diseases. For instance, both Linus Pauling in his book "Cancer and Vitamin C," and William Boyd in his book "A Textbook Of Pathology" (which is one of the most widely used textbooks of its kind,) point out that cancer of the prostate is found in almost fifty percent of older men. Yet it seldom develops further and becomes symptomatic, *as the body's immune system keeps it in check.* Dr. Ernest T. Krebs, Jr. believes that many people have undiagnosed cancer in the course of their lives. The reason why this goes unnoticed in the majority of cases is because *the body's immune system can easily destroy these early malignancies if it is functioning normally.* More recently,

Sir MacFarlane Burnet, Nobel prize winner for his work in immunology, judged that 100,000 cells can become cancerous in the body each day. *But, if the immune system is functioning normally, it effectively destroys these cancer cells.*

If the above is true, then only about one cancer in twenty, or perhaps even less, develops further and becomes life-threatening.

The average age of cancer patients is another factor which points to the important role played by the immune system in this condition. Statistics show that cancer occurs most frequently in the very young and the very old, that is, at ages when the immune system has either not had time to develop fully, or it has become weakened because of age. Middle-aged individuals develop cancer comparatively infrequently since the body's resistance is strongest between the ages of approximately twenty and fifty-five.

The fact that irritation is the only specific cause of cancer has been known since scientific studies of this condition began. Carcinogens are entities which sufficiently irritate the body so as to cause cancer.

The most obvious examples of the role played by irritants (carcinogens) are cancers of the skin and lungs. It is a well established fact that skin cancer is usually the result of excessive exposure to the sun or some other external irritant. For example, city cab drivers frequently get cancer on the left arm, which is the one exposed to the sun. Chimney sweeps formerly developed skin cancer to an alarming degree because of irritation caused by soot.

Everybody knows that lung cancer can be caused by chronic irritation of the tissues of the lungs as a result of smoking or exposure to irritants in the air—smoke from cigarettes smoked by others, dust, fumes, etc. Cigarette smoking became popular in the 1920's. About thirty years later we felt the results. Thousands of men and women began dying of lung cancer.

In Sweden, doctors have been treating cancer patients successfully for a long time by placing them on an intermittent water fast. As with all the other natural approaches to cancer, the main purpose of this fast is to cleanse the body and strengthen the immune system. The patients are allowed only distilled water on some days of the fast while on other days they can also eat fresh, organically grown fruits.

From these stories it can be seen that cancer is far from the killer we have been taught to believe. In fact, it is likely that one day science will discover that cancer is not a disease at all, but only a last ditch attempt on the part of the body to protect itself from irritation.

As long as the body's resistance is strong, it can protect itself easily from irritants. When the immune system breaks down, the body can no longer cope with the effects of the irritant (carcinogen). Therefore, it tries to protect itself by throwing up a barricade of rapidly dividing cells. Since this mass of cells, or tumor, is the only visible sign of the condition, we have mistakenly interpreted it as being the disease itself and given it the name "cancer".

If the chronic irritation ceases, the barricade of cancer cells is no longer necessary and the body soon removes it. No one ever died from cancer. "Cancer" patients die of extreme toxicity and a breakdown of the immune system. Many examples of this are discussed in Dr. Max Gerson's book, "A Cancer Therapy, Results Of Fifty Cases." The main purpose of the Gerson treatment is to strengthen the immune system and cleanse the body of irritating toxins. This is done with the help of fresh juices, enemas, and other natural means. Dr. Gerson was successful in saving the lives of many terminally ill cancer patients who had been given up by orthodox doctors. Many of the patients whose stories are told in Dr. Gerson's book only had days to live when his treatment was started. They had massive tumors all over their bodies and there appeared to be no hope left. Yet they promptly recovered when their immune system became stronger and the irritation ceased when their bodies were cleansed of toxins.

Here we have the same picture as in the cases mentioned earlier. The stories in Dr. Gerson's book clearly show that cancer is not a disease in itself. So-called malignant tumors are only a sign that the body has become too weak to cope with the carcinogen. When the toxic irritant is removed and the immune system recovers, the body soon heals itself.

One of the best documented examples of the effectiveness of natural methods in the treatment of cancer is that of Dr. Anthony Sattilaro. In his book, "Recalled By Life," Dr. Sattilaro describes how he was diagnosed as having numerous malignant tumors throughout his body—

his skull, ribs, pelvis, spine, and prostate. As could be expected, three surgeries and hormone therapy only made matters much worse. The patient became weak, bloated and depressed. Even the best specialists gave him no hope for recovery. Ironically, Dr. Sattilaro's life was saved by a young hippy who was thumbing a lift on a freeway. By following the macrobiotic diet suggested by his new friend, the first person to give him hope, Dr. Sattilaro soon cured his cancer. (A brief description of the macrobiotic diet will be given later in this book.)

Great advances have also been made in homeopathy since electro-diagnosis has made it easier to discover which homeopathic remedies should be used. Homeopathic remedies have been used successfully in the treatment of cancer for a long time. As early as 1929, Dr. A. H. Grimmer wrote in the Homeopathic Recorder:

> The curing of cancer cases with homeopathic remedies is nothing new or strange.... In the past four years I have treated two hundred and twenty-five cases of various forms and in all stages of the disease. At this time one hundred and seventy-five are still living, many of them entirely well and free of all cancer symptoms. Only one of this group shows indications of an early demise. All of those who failed to respond to the homeopathic treatment had been treated surgically or with X-ray and radium in material doses.

Recently, homeopathic remedies have been developed in Europe which detoxify the body with incredible effectiveness. As a result, those cases of cancer which can be treated in the early stages of the disease, can be cured in a short time. The problem with the more advanced cases is that the weakened patient may find it difficult to eliminate large tumors and accumulations of toxins from the body. Unless these cases follow a very strict diet, under the supervision of an experienced physician, the prognosis may remain uncertain for some time.

It is also essential that the patient eliminate all toxic influences from his environment. At some of the European cancer clinics doctors insist that patients wear only clothing made of cotton and wool. The use of cosmetics and even the wearing of watches, rings, and other jewelry is not allowed. Chemicals, sprays, deodorants, hair bleaches, etc., are never used. Electro-diagnosis provides an ideal, quick means of checking for harmful reactions and eliminating damaging influences.

The speed with which patients recover under these natural conditions is truly amazing. Tumors diminish in size so rapidly that the difference can be noticed from one day to the next. Even seemingly hopeless cases often recover.

Two other successful treatments for cancer are those developed by Dr. William Kelley and Dr. Virginia Livingstone-Wheeler. Like all other doctors who use natural methods for the treatment of cancer, these physicians also stress the importance of cleansing the body and strengthening the immune system. The main difference is that Dr. Livingstone-Wheeler also uses a vaccine to fight bacteria, which she says are always present in the body but become invasive in cancer patients. In her book, "The Conquest Of Cancer," she quotes many case histories of terminal cancer patients who were successfully treated at her clinic in San Diego, California.

On the other hand, Dr. Kelley recommended taking large quantities of pancreatic enzymes to help detoxify and cleanse the cancer patient's body. He believes that cancer is only a symptom of a diminished pancreatic enzyme production, in a similar way that diabetes is only a symptom of insufficient insulin being produced by the pancreas. When the pancreas does not produce sufficient enzymes, one of whose functions Dr. Kelley says is to remove toxins from the tissues, excessive poisons accumulate in some areas and cancer may develop. Dr. Kelley has written two excellent books entitled "One Answer To Cancer" and "Dr. Kelley's Answer To Cancer."

Of the vitamins which have been used successfully in the treatment of cancer, the best known of these are Vitamin A, Vitamin C, and of course, Vitamin B-17 or Laetrile. The supporters of Laetrile suggest that a lack of this vitamin in the diet could be the main reason why cancer develops in the first place. They point out that in Hunza, whose inhabitants consume a diet high in Vitamin B-17, cancer does not exist.

A number of excellent books have been written about Laetrile. The best of these are "World Without Cancer," by G. Edward Griffin, "The Death of Cancer," by Dr. Harold W. Manner, and "An End To Cancer? The Nutritional

Approach to its Prevention and Control," by Leon Chaitow, N.D., D.O. No one should miss reading these three wonderfully written and most informative books.

Laetrile is being used with great success in many European countries as well as the Mexican cancer clinics. To the despair of its advocates the use of Laetrile is prohibited by law in the United States. This is not because Laetrile is useless or dangerous in any way, but because organized medicine has to protect itself from all possible competition while it experiments with its favorite cut, burn and poison therapies. While Laetrile has been used successfully to help numerous patients back to health, these invasive therapies have exterminated more Americans than all the wars this country has ever taken part in. However, this fact has been conveniently overlooked by the establishment.

The discovery of electro-diagnosis as a diagnostic tool is the most significant recent advancement in the field of cancer prevention and treatment. This method of diagnosis has given us a much broader understanding of the causes of cancer. In the past, successful cancer cures depended primarily on detoxifying the patient's body and strengthening his immune system. This was done by using natural diets, vitamins, fresh juices, enemas, etc. Since electro-diagnosis has been used, it has finally become clear why detoxifying programs cannot always be successful by themselves in saving cancer patient's lives—some patients are still succumbing to the dread disease even if they appear to improve initially.

Electro-diagnosis has shown that there are a great number of other factors which can cause abnormal changes in the body's chemistry. Unless these problems are also corrected, it may be impossible to cure a cancer patient even if a very strict diet and cleansing program are conscientiously followed. These factors include: toxic materials used in dentistry, intestinal parasites (worms, Giardia, yeasts,) residual sensitivities to previous infections (whether symptoms were present or not,) traces of pesticides in the tissues, certain preservatives, chemicals, cosmetics and deodorants, etc.—in short, all those factors which cause abnormal changes to occur in the body's electromagnetic field and interfere with the normal flow of energy along the meridians.

In many cases, the most important of the above factors are (1) intestinal parasites, (2) toxic chemicals and (3) the toxic materials (metals, acrylics, and cements) used in dentistry. In Germany it has been found that correcting only these three problems is often enough to turn the tide. When a patient is cleansed of intestinal parasites and toxic chemicals, and all harmful materials are removed from his teeth, the toxic load is sufficiently reduced to allow his body to begin healing itself.

When one learns more about cancer and reads the available literature, one cannot help wondering how such killers as chemotherapy, radiation and surgery could have ever become the only accepted "therapies of choice" for treating cancer. These treatments are entirely symptom-oriented and do nothing to correct the cause of the problem.

In fact, they are the best known ways of weakening the body further and making it even more difficult for the cancer patient to recover.

No wonder that after a study which took over twenty years, Dr. Hardin Jones, Professor of Medical Physics and Physiology at Berkeley, California found that women with breast cancer survived four times longer without conventional treatments. Women who refused treatment lived for an average of twelve and a half years while those who submitted to orthodox treatments lived an average of only three years. In other words, conventional methods for treating cancer shortened the lives of these patients by an average of nine and a half years!

By using the most unnatural forms of treatment they can find, Western doctors have transformed cancer into a monster. A condition which in itself is little more that a symptom of extreme toxicity has been promoted to the status of the most feared disease of modern times. The therapies used on cancer patients do not strengthen their bodies so they can better cope with the cancer. They weaken the patients and make it even more difficult for them to recover. Cancer patients are exterminated, or, if you prefer, slowly tortured to death by well-meaning doctors who do not know what they are doing.

On the other hand, the wonderful results obtained with the use of homeopathy and other natural methods, which show a success rate of over 90 percent in the case of beginning cancers, have had no effect on Western medical thinking. This is true even though the results obtained with natural methods have been improved dramatically since electro-diagnostic instruments have made diagnosis easier. Chemotherapy, radiation and surgery are still being used, regardless of the fact that statistics show the long term success rate to be negligible. Common sense tells us that no one can possibly be helped by such murderous procedures. They have to make everyone they are used on much worse, even if initially there is an illusion of temporary improvement.

This tragic situation has arisen because of the indisputable fact that Western methods for treating cancer do destroy tumors. Dazzled by the sight of tumors melting away under radiation and chemotherapy, doctors have overlooked the obvious fact that the main problem is not the tumors themselves but a rundown immune system and toxicity. Orthodox methods result in still greater weakness and even more pollution of the body. They can do nothing but make matters worse except in some rare cases where, if used very judiciously, they may be helpful in speeding up the breakdown of tumors which happen to be pressing on vital structures or organs.

Statistics prove that we are making no headway whatsoever. In 1971, the year that President Nixon signed the National Cancer Act, which marked the beginning of the war against cancer, the disease killed 350,000 Americans. Since then this figure has increased steadily and is now approaching half a million cancer deaths per year. The following quotation from an article in the 1986 summer issue of the magazine, "The Choice," confirms this gloomy statement:

U.S. medical orthodoxy was stunned in May of 1986 by the analysis in the prestigious New England Journal of Medicine which showed that the nation's multi-billion-dollar "war on cancer" has failed, that the overall death rates are worse than ever and that more money and energy should be put into prevention.

No one can deny that modern medicine has been miraculously successful in helping patients with life-threatening conditions. Many people on the brink of death have been sensationally helped with surgery, drugs and other modern crisis therapies. However, this great success has had an unfortunate side effect. Doctors have become afflicted with a sort of tunnel vision. The same therapies which have proved themselves to be successful in treating patients with critical problems are being used as the only valid treatments for practically all ailments. Even in the face of the most hopeless failures, modern medicine is obstinately trying to adapt its crisis therapies to chronic conditions. Cancer is one of the best examples. After so many years and millions of dollars spent for negligible results, it is still assumed that the cure for cancer will be a chemical or some other ingenious medical discovery, which will kill malignant cells without harming healthy ones.

This kind of thinking has resulted in the greatest tragedy in the history of medicine. Millions upon millions of lives have been lost or ruined unnecessarily. Chemotherapy, radiation and surgery simply cannot be used successfully for treating cancer. Only natural therapies can be effective.

Unfortunately, Western medicine seems to be willing to accept only those remedies or solutions for cancer which it can fully control. This way, doctors can pose as the only ones who understand what is being done. Since natural methods cannot be monopolized, and they can be easily understood by the patient, they are automatically condemned. Every effort is made to prevent this route of healing from being used, no matter how much better it may be than the so-called proven therapies.

Besides, doctors have an aversion to anything natural. The vile thought of having to treat patients with carrot juice and enemas makes them shudder with revulsion. They would not feel superior and educated. In fact they would no longer feel like real doctors at all.

Modern medicine views Nature itself as a dangerous competitor. So no one can attribute a patient's recovery to the healing power of Nature, hospitals are transformed into the most unnatural places possible. Patients are not encouraged to choose wholesome foods which would promote healing and build up the immune system. Instead they have to subsist on the most artificial junk foods, full of preservatives, additives, refined white sugar and white flour products—like airline food at its worst. There are rancid fatty meats and sugary sweets for breakfast, lunch and dinner. What vegetables are offered are cooked until the last trace of life has been boiled out of them. Anyone who has seen hospital food might easily make the mistake of concluding that the hospital is deliberately trying to prevent the patients from getting better.

None of the elements which promote health—fresh air and sunshine, fresh fruits and vegetables, vitamins, etc.—can be found anywhere in a hospital. No wonder that, when doctors go on strike the death rates drop. For instance, in 1973, doctors in Israel reduced their patient contact from 65,000 to 7,000 for a period of one month because of a doctor's strike. During that time the death rate dropped by fifty percent.

It took over a hundred years to convince surgeons that they should wash their hands before entering the operating room. We will probably have to wait another hundred years before doctors finally become reconciled to the necessity of having to use natural therapies when treating chronic conditions.

It seems that it is all a matter of trying to stay in control. Organized medicine simply cannot stand the thought that someone else could have any power over the patient, or that the patient should take any responsibility for his own recovery. That this has been the case since the beginning of time can be seen from a rather comical complaint by a Byzantine doctor of the early fifth century. He wrote:

> As the patient lies on his bed prostrated by the severity of the disease, there quickly comes into the room a crowd of us physicians. No feeling of sympathy for the sick man have we, nor do we realize how impotent we are in the presence of those forces of nature. Instead, we struggle to the best of our ability to obtain charge of the case: one depending for success on his powers of persuasion

the second on the strength of the arguments he is able to bring forward, the third on his readiness to agree with everything that is said, and the fourth on his skill in contradicting the opinions of everybody else.

In the midst of this struggle for control, the patient and his interests may easily be forgotten.

Another reason why organized medicine is finding it hard to make any headway is the fear of malpractice suits. If a patient dies under the care of a doctor who is using "accepted therapies" a suit cannot be brought against him. The treatment he is using may be useless, or it may even kill the patient, but it is "accepted." Therefore, in case of trouble, the doctor can count on the support of other doctors and specialists. But if the doctor tries to use a new treatment, he cannot count on support in case of failure. Medical malpractice suits do more harm than good. They should be prohibited by law.

Most people treat their bodies the same way they treat their automobile. They show little interest until something goes wrong. When that happens, they go to their doctor expecting him to fix things quickly, so they can carry on as before. Although this system does work part of the time, it is not always the best way to go. If you spend a little time each week studying health books, you will soon discover that there are many easy things you can do to improve your health and prevent chronic diseases, especially cancer. The books listed at the end of the introduction are especially useful in this respect. Most of them can be found in public libraries or health food stores.

"There Is A Cure For Arthritis," by Paavo Airola, is probably the most relevant of these health books. Like cancer, rheumatoid arthritis is also caused by the body becoming overloaded with toxins. As in the case of cancer, doctors have no cure for rheumatoid arthritis. While conventional treatments do give some temporary relief, in the long run they only make matters much worse. Paavo Airola describes how, when treated at European health clinics with natural methods, even the most hopelessly crippled arthritic patients soon recovered.

Cancer, and many other chronic conditions can also be treated successfully, but only with natural therapies. When our doctors learn to understand and use natural methods, cancer will cease to exist, and so will many other chronic conditions.

At present, since most Western doctors do not want to use natural therapies, cancer patients just have to go on dying, and rheumatoid arthritis sufferers have to continue putting up with their sufferings. There is no hope for either, at least not until natural treatments become accepted.

SUMMARY

Whether in preventing cancer or curing it, the most important steps to take are: (1) identify the causes of interference with the energy flow along the meridian system of your body, (2) strengthen your immune system and (3) cleanse your body of unwanted toxins.

With the help of electro-diagnosis and muscle-testing, it is possible not only to detect cancer in its earliest stages, but also determine exactly what caused your body to break down so the malignancy could develop in the first place.

In the past, Western doctors were handicapped by their inability to diagnose patients' conditions with sufficient accuracy. The commonly used diagnostic procedures had two serious flaws. They were seldom able to detect problems before obvious symptoms appeared, and they gave no clues as to the causes of the disorder. As a result, doctors were often reduced to treating only symptoms. They had no understanding of the underlying causes of even the simplest and most common health problems.

One can only imagine what would happen if our doctors, like the Chinese doctors, were paid only as long as their patients remained well and had to treat them for nothing if they became sick. With the exception of some procedures which are now used successfully in crisis situations, the rest of modern medicine would disappear into thin air—which would be so much the worse for the drug companies and so much the better for everyone else. Although modern diagnostic procedures do have some limited value in emergency situations, they are practically worthless if they have to be used for the prevention of health problems. Although billions have been spent on attempts to discover useless miracle cures, almost no research has been done on how common problems could be prevented.

Warning: It is dangerous to attempt fasts without professional supervision. If you wish to follow some of the recommendations mentioned in this book, you should do so only with the help and advice of competent medical assistance.

4   Amalgam—A Poison In Your Mouth

Many European researchers now believe that the highly toxic materials used in dentistry are an important, if not the most important, reason for the cancer epidemic of modern times. This is largely because there are many well-documented cases of terminal cancer patients who recovered only when the toxic materials, mainly amalgam and nickel, were removed from their teeth. Before that, all therapies which were used on these people failed.

The amalgam scare has been gaining momentum for some time. This is because silver (amalgam) fillings contain fifty percent mercury, one of the most toxic and poisonous metals. Silver fillings were thought to be safe in the past mainly because very few patients showed an immediate allergic reaction to amalgam. If a person started having symptoms later, the relationship of the disorder to the silver fillings was hard to prove. There were no tests sensitive enough to detect the effects amalgam fillings have on the body. Since amalgam is very durable and easy to handle, it was conveniently assumed that it was safe. For some unknown reason, most dentists stubbornly insisted that all evidence unfavorable to amalgam was unscientific and inconclusive. The few dentists who tried to warn their patients of the dangers of amalgam toxicity were even threatened with the loss of their licenses.

Since electro-diagnosis and muscle-testing have made diagnosis more accurate, it has been possible to prove clearly the hazards presented by silver fillings.

These new methods of diagnosis have shown that:

1. Everyone, with no exception, shows a strong sensitivity to amalgam.
2. Even the smallest quantities of amalgam can cause serious interference with the energy flow in the body.
3. Amalgam fillings can cause abnormal changes in the body's electromagnetic field.
4. When the amalgam is removed from the teeth, traces of mercury can still be found in the brain, kidneys, and other tissues. ALWAYS!
5. The tissues close to the amalgam fillings remain chronically inflamed, all the time, from the moment of insertion.

Another important effect amalgam has is that it can seriously depress the immune system. For instance, in an article entitled "Amalgam Toxicity: Grand Deception," Dr. Victor Penzer D.D.S. writes:

In the pilot research by Eggleston, as reported in the *Journal Of Prosthetic Dentistry*, two patients with depressed lymphocytes, had amalgams replaced with temporary fillings, and the T-lymphocyte count went up. When the amalgams were experimentally reinserted the T-lymphocytes dropped again. They improved once more when the amalgams were eliminated.

T-lymphocytes are white blood cells whose function is to fight infection and remove toxic elements from the tissues. The number of T-lymphocytes in the blood reflects the body's ability to fight invasion. From the above experiment it can be seen that amalgam can immediately depress the immune system.

The damaging effects of amalgams are often largely due to the interference they cause with the flow of energy along the meridian system. Therefore, the symptoms a person develops depend on which part of this system is affected most. In Germany, Doctors Voll and Thompson have mapped the relationship of each tooth to certain organs, muscles, and joints. They have found that if an amalgam filling or some other toxic material is placed in a tooth, a specific area of the body will be affected. This happens because the toxic fillings interfere with the energy flow to that part of the body, and this results in immediate malfunction.

We have become so accustomed to accepting a second class state of health as the norm, that sickness has become an accepted part of life for many people. If you ask these people whether they ever have headaches, indigestion, insomnia, depression, fatigue, irritability, backaches, or other aches and pains, they will look at you in surprise and say something like, "No more than usual! I am really lucky, I enjoy very good health!" It never crossed their minds that such symptoms could be caused by the toxic materials their dentist placed in their teeth.

In the process of gathering material for this book, I have spoken to a great many people who had their amalgams replaced with non-toxic materials. Most of them reported significant improvements in health. The symptoms which cleared up, after the amalgams and other toxic materials were removed from the teeth of these individuals, included: cancer, headaches, joint pains, backaches, fatigue, indigestion, menstrual cramps, hair loss, inability to concentrate, fits of rage, hemorrhoids, bad breath, arthritic pain, weakness, trembling, paralysis, enlarged lymph nodes in the neck, migraines, etc. Dr. Max Garten, the author of several books on health, even told me that two of his patients who had been diagnosed as having multiple sclerosis recovered and were able to get out of their wheelchairs when their amalgams were removed. Leading homeopaths in Germany, who use electro-diagnosis, believe that close to ninety percent of the time, multiple sclerosis is caused by toxic materials placed in patients' teeth by dentists.

Recently candidiasis, a yeast overgrowth, has attracted a great deal of attention. This condition has also been linked to amalgam fillings. There appears to be a connection between the presence of amalgam in the teeth and the body's ability to resist the yeast, candida albicans. When the immune system is weakened, candida can multiply until it produces disease-like symptoms—such as aching joints, swelling, bloating, fatigue, headaches, etc. Removal of the amalgam fillings often produces a marked improvement in the symptoms caused by candida.

In Germany some of the leading holistic doctors refuse to treat patients who have amalgams in their teeth. They know that no treatment can be fully effective unless the toxic fillings are removed.

Amalgam is by no means the only toxic material dentists use on unsuspecting patients. There are many others. The most dangerous of these is probably nickel. In a lecture given at the Holistic Dental Convention in 1983, Dr. David Eggleston had this to say about nickel:

Nickel is used routinely by national cancer centers to induce cancer in laboratory animals to study cancer. The nickel alloys they are using are very similar to those we are using in patients' mouths. Dentists are causing a major health problem.

Dr. Harold Kristal, D.D.S., whose practice is in Point Richmond near San Francisco, has done some of the most outstanding work on the problem of amalgam toxicity. In a talk on this subject Dr. Kristal said:

"There are five ways in which mercury, from amalgam restorations, spreads throughout the body. (1) About 76 percent of all vapors that exude from mercury fillings upon chewing are inhaled into the lungs. (2) Particles of silver fillings that break off when we chew are swallowed and pass into the digestive tract. (3) If a silver filling happens to be close to the gum line, the mercury seeps directly into the arteries and veins. It then spreads throughout the body. (4) The mercury is absorbed through the dental tubules into the pulp arteriovenous system. It then spreads throughout the body. (5) The fifth and last way that mercury is transmitted to different parts of the body is though the nervous system. The vapors are absorbed into the Trigeminal and Olfactory nerves and pass along these nerves to the brain. The mercury will travel approximately ten millimeters a day along the nerve tract until it reaches the brain. This is very frightening because the simple vaporization from mercury can create various problems with brain function.

This work was brought up by Dr. Patrick Stortebecker, M.D., Ph.D., a researcher in Sweden. His book is called "Mercury poisoning From Dental Amalgams—A Hazard To The Human Brain." Dr. Stortebecker's work is very outstanding. He feels that many of the problems that we are having in our culture today are primarily brought about by the 150 years of mercury poisoning that has been thrust upon the human race. If you add this to the complex pollution that exists in the atmosphere today, together with other pollutants, you can begin to see the enormity of the problem.

It is felt that during the chewing process a person with an average of only three to five amalgams, may reach perhaps 10 to 100 times the toxic mercury levels that O.S.H.A. approves in ambient air in their various working places. Many people have as many as ten amalgams and in some cases many more.

I would now like to discuss nickel. Nickel is not nearly as active as mercury, however, it corrodes and is far more carcinogenic. The corrosion of these non-precious metals into the gum tissues, and then into the blood, creates tremendous havoc for millions of people.

One of the most severe known reactions to nickel toxicity is described by Dr. Eggleston. A patient presented herself to the Long Beach Memorial Hospital with kidney disease. She was diagnosed as having idiopathic glomerulo-nephritis. They called it idiopathic because they did not know what was really the cause of the kidney ailment. After examining the patient, her family physician suggested that she be checked with electro-diagnosis. When this was done it was found that she was highly reactive to nickel. The doctor asked her if she had any dental work done within the past seven years. She said that she had three porcelain crowns put in by her dentist. The doctor explained that porcelain crowns have metal jackets (made of a nickel alloy) underneath the porcelain and suggested that she have these crowns removed immediately. After the removal of the three crowns the patient lost all symptoms of kidney failure. This was one case in a million which was diagnosed properly. Her kidney problem was primarily due to the nickel toxicity. This was poisoning her system.

I would now like to relate another case that I had myself. This patient had cancer surgery and had her breast removed in 1977. She came to me in late 1978 and I removed all her amalgam fillings. The only remaining restorations were seven nickel crowns in the front portion of her upper mouth. In 1984, when it became clear that nickel is a causative agent in cancer, I suggested to her that we should remove these seven crowns. However, before this was done a very exacting immunological checkup was performed. Six months after all seven crowns were removed, I did another immunological testing on her. To my great surprise I found that her complete immune system had strengthened amazingly. She had twice as many T-cells, twice the number of T-8 cells, and a much better balance of T-4 and T-8 cells. Her B cells also increased. In general, it is felt that if she had those nickel crowns removed earlier she might have had the immune system to fight and ward off the cancer.

I would like to describe another case that I had. A patient of mine, aged 65, was suffering from rheumatoid arthritis. She had a lower partial which was made primarily of nickel and cobalt. She had one tiny mercury filling in her lower teeth. This patient had only six lower teeth left, the rest were dentures. Full upper denture and this lower partial which was made of nickel and cobalt. I immediately removed the small mercury filling she had and changed her partial to a gold partial. Shortly after this was done she no longer had to take pain medication. She was on nine Tylenols a day. Even the mobility in her joints improved somewhat. This patient said that she traces the beginning of her rheumatoid arthritis to the insertion of that partial twenty-five years earlier.

I would like to describe one last patient of mine who has been with me since he was a little boy. Four years ago he came to me complaining of severe back pains and cramping in his legs, which made it impossible for him to do any physical work. He ran a large company and his restrictions presented a major problem. He said that he was going to many rheumatologists. They thought he had some kind of arthritis, but they did not know which kind. To be able to function, he had to take strong pain killers during the day. If he did not he was unable to get out of bed and he could not get any work done.

I checked his teeth with electro-diagnosis and found him to be very sensitive to both mercury and nickel. I had used both of these materials in his mouth ten or fifteen years earlier. Upon finding this I suggested that we remove all these restorations and replace them with gold and composites. We did this and two weeks later he lost all pain. I can hardly wait for the day when these materials are banned in this country."

Toxic materials, such as mercury or nickel, play an important part in disrupting normal function. By checking materials—metals, acrylics, cements, porcelains, etc.—with electro-diagnosis, it is now possible to determine which of them cause allergic reactions and which do not. You should make certain that all materials used by your dentist are carefully checked before they are permanently installed in your teeth. Only amalgam and nickel have been mentioned here, since they are by far the most toxic and dangerous materials used by dentists. However, some persons have been found to exhibit a strong sensitivity to many of the other materials used in dental restorations. You should make certain that your dentist checks everything he puts in your teeth with electro-diagnosis—gold, platinum, porcelain, cements, acrylics, composites, etc. Nothing should be permanently inserted in your teeth without first being carefully checked. For instance, you cannot "assume" that gold is O.K. It may not be. A leading homeopath once told me the story of a medical doctor who became violently ill and developed seizures because he was sensitive to the gold crowns in his mouth.

In his book, "*Naked Empress—Or The Great Medical Fraud*," Hans Ruesch explains that, because of the frequency of drug reactions and other complications which can result from medical treatments, modern medicine has become a leading cause of health complications in civilized countries. There may be some truth in that statement, but Hans Ruesch has overlooked dentists. Dentists cause infinitely more trouble. The toxic materials used in dentistry have a chronic debilitating effect on health. They act like road blocks on the body's energy pathways and make normal energy flow an impossibility. Everyone who has toxic materials in his mouth has to have health problems of one kind or another. They just don't realize it. Most people have become so accustomed to "normal headaches" and "normal fatigue" and "normal complaints" of different kinds, that they no longer know whether they are sick or not. They have never been truly well so they cannot compare their present state of health to anything tangible.

Amalgam and The Thyroid

Since muscle-testing has begun to be used an unusual discovery has been made concerning the apparent effects of amalgam fillings on the thyroid gland. Muscle-testing has shown that even the smallest traces of mercury in the body seem to cause serious thyroid weakness.

Muscle-testing is perhaps most useful when nutritional deficiencies have to be detected. By using this method it is possible to not only discover what deficiencies of vitamins and minerals a person has, but also precisely how much of each nutritional supplement should be taken.

When muscle-testing is used to check for supplements made of animal thyroid, most people show some need for this form of nutritional help. However, there is a great difference between those persons who have amalgam fillings, or even the slightest traces of mercury in their body, and persons who are found to have no mercury contamination whatsoever. Those who have no mercury usually show only a very slight need for animal thyroid tablets. They may need just one or two tablets at the most, which presumably means that their thyroid is strong and needs little help. But persons who have amalgam fillings react differently. They always show a need for a very large amount of thyroid, often more than thirty or even forty tablets. But when all the amalgam is taken out of their teeth and all the mercury is removed from their tissues (this can be accomplished with homeopathic remedies or with a soft laser), their need for thyroid supplementation immediately drops drastically, usually to only one or two tablets.

For some time, certain researchers have believed that hypothyroidism (a thyroid weakness) plays an important part in causing cancer. For example, in a lecture given to the International Academy of Preventive Medicine in Texas, Samuel Schwartz, M.D., presented his work, "The Incidence of Cancer in Patients with Thyroid Dysfunction". He pointed out that in his observation ALL of his patients who were diagnosed as hypothyroid (with below normal thyroid function) and were untreated, eventually developed cancer, within eight to twenty years. On the other hand, ALL who were treated (i.e. given supplemental thyroid), and remained on the treatment program, had NO incidence of cancer. Dr. Schwartz also stated that hyperthyroid (over active thyroid) patients seldom, if ever, develop cancer.

Could this mean that everyone who has silver amalgam fillings, and consequent thyroid weakness, has to develop cancer? Unless they happen to die of something else first.

Nickel And The Pancreas

Thanks to the use of muscle-testing an interesting discovery has also been made regarding the effect of nickel on the pancreas. Muscle-testing has shown that if a nickel object comes in contact with the body this appears to severely depress pancreatic function. Those persons who have dental restorations made of alloys containing nickel, or who wear jewelry made of nickel alloys, show a tremendous need for pancreatic enzymes when muscle-tested. They are often found to need as many as fifty or even sixty tablets of animal pancreas. On the other hand, those who do not have nickel interfering with the flow of energy in their bodies are found to need either very little or no pancreatic enzyme supplementation.

As already mentioned earlier in this book, some researchers believe that cancer is a symptom of pancreatic dysfunction. They believe that pancreatic enzymes do not just help digest the food in the small intestine, but they are also carried, in the blood, to all parts of the body to help breakup and remove waste matter. If insufficient pancreatic enzymes are available, the accumulations of wastes become so great that eventually cancerous tumors may begin to form. In other words, in the same way that diabetes is caused by the pancreas not producing enough insulin, cancer is a symptom the pancreas is not manufacturing enough enzymes. This may explain why nickel has such a strong carcinogenic effect and why nickel implants cause the rapid growth of tumors in experimental animals.

Now that the harmful effects of nickel and mercury are better understood, many leading European holistic doctors consider that the removal of these toxic metals is essential if treatment is to be successful. This is because they have found that merely the removal of these toxic metals is often enough to dramatically help some patients. Not only have many cancer patients spontaneously recovered when the toxic metals were removed from their teeth, but many other patients with serious chronic conditions—multiple sclerosis, rheumatoid arthritis, debilitating migraine headaches, chronic fatigue, etc.—have also been helped. The following testimonials written by patients who travelled from the United States to be treated by these German doctors are good examples of the success of this approach.

1. "At age forty-two I noticed a small lump on the back of my head. This did not go away and after a few months began to fester and bleed frequently. When I washed my hair I often noticed a speck of blood on the towel. When I went in for my annual checkup I told my doctor about the lump and asked him if there was something he could do about it. After examining it he told me there was little doubt in his mind that I had a malignant tumor on my head known as a "melanoma" because of its dark color. He said it was the most dangerous form of cancer known and advised me to see a specialist as soon as possible. Many examinations followed and I saw not one but several specialists. The prognosis they gave me differed. One doctor told me that I could have only a few months to live, while another said I could live as long as five years, although statistics showed the chance of that happening was very slim indeed. The one thing that all the specialists agreed on was that if I wanted to prolong my life I should start treatment as soon as possible. This was to consist of a three pronged attack: radiation, chemotherapy and surgery to remove the lymph nodes in

my neck and in my armpits. The doctors assured me I was dealing with the most deadly variety of cancer and said there was no time to lose. Delay could be fatal and my only chance was the immediate commencement of aggressive therapy. I feared they were right because it so happened that only a year previously our neighbor's son, who was only nineteen at the time, also developed the same disease. He had a melanoma on his arm and soon after this was removed surgically the cancer appeared in other parts of his body. He was dead within nine months. The doctor told the parents that it was a miracle he had lived so long and that he would probably have lived only six months, or even less, had it not been for the vigorous chemotherapy treatment which had prolonged his life, as well as removing every hair on his body and changing his appearance to that of a walking skeleton. The thought of this poor boy terrified me and I was very open to trying any alternative treatment. It so happened that at that very time my wife, who was going to a holistic doctor for treatment, came home with news of the wonderful success German homeopathic doctors were having with cancer patients. After listening to what she had to say, I decided to go to Germany, and only submit to conventional therapies if everything else failed. We called a German doctor who had been recommended to us and got an appointment for seventeen days later. This was the earliest he could see me. The following day, on the advice of the German doctor, I went to a dentist, who had been recommended to me as having experience in this procedure, to have all my fillings and crowns removed and replaced with non-toxic composites. On the advice of a friend, who had been reading Michio Kushi's book *The Cancer Prevention Diet* and other books on cleansing, I also started on the macrobiotic diet, as well as taking large amounts of garlic to kill any parasites and fungal organisms. When I went to see the German doctor he examined me with his electro-diagnostic instrument and gave me a number of different homeopathic remedies which I was to take after my return to the U.S. He felt my cancer was already under control and would never return. This, in fact, turned out to be the case. Following my trip to Germany my health improved steadily. Six years have passed since my cancer was discovered and there has been no recurrence. I no longer have any fear of dying of cancer. I feel that cancer is a disease which can be easily prevented if one follows a healthful life-style and avoids habits which cause the body to become overloaded with poisons.

2. "My health had been deteriorating steadily for the past ten years. I had daily headaches, fatigue, and almost constant low grade back pain and stiffness. If I remained in the same position for any length of time I would become so stiff that movement was difficult. The simple act of turning over in bed had

become a major problem, as had getting out of bed. After sleeping I was so stiff and in so much pain that it would take me half an hour before I could move reasonably comfortably. When I was fifty-two my doctor told me that I had prostate cancer and should go in for immediate surgery to try and prevent the cancer from spreading. Fearing that I could have cancer, I had been reading some books on this subject. I had become interested in the German cancer clinics since a friend of mine had been successfully treated there. The German doctors had been able to solve the problem of her cancer very quickly when all other approaches she had tried failed. Encouraged by my friend I made an appointment with a German doctor for the earliest available date. When I arrived in Germany I went straight to the clinic from the airport. The doctor examined me with an electro-diagnostic instrument and after prescribing some homeopathic remedies he advised me to remove all mercury fillings and restorations containing nickel from my teeth. He also said that I had traces of cadmium in my tissues and advised some homeopathic remedies for removing them. He said that cadmium is a highly carcinogenic metal and unless this was removed it could cause a return of the cancer. The German doctor seemed confident that I would get well, without surgery, and said that the cancer would not return if the toxic metals were removed and if I ate a healthful diet and avoided certain foods he had found me to be sensitive to. Eight years have passed since my visit to Germany and I have had no recurrence of the cancer or any of my previous problems. I no longer have headaches or back pain and, what I find most amazing, all the stiffness has disappeared. The most noticeable improvement occurred when my porcelain crowns were removed. The German doctor said they had to be taken out because they had metal jackets made of an alloy containing nickel. He told me that I need have no fear of a return of the cancer as long as I keep my body reasonably free of toxins. He also advised me to follow a healthful diet and exercise regularly to keep my immune system strong. The doctor told me that cancer is only a symptom of toxicity and a weak immune system. It occurs in people who abuse their bodies by drinking, smoking, eating junk foods and not exercising regularly."

3. "When I was thirty-two I began suffering with chronic abdominal pains which would sometimes keep me awake at night. When the pain would not stop I eventually went to my doctor to see if he could help me. At first he thought it was simple indigestion, but when the medication he gave me did not help he decided to run some tests and sent me to a hospital for a more thorough examination. Suspecting that something more serious could be wrong, the doctors at the hospital decided to perform exploratory surgery and found numerous can-

cerous tumors. They said they were afraid to remove them for fear that I would bleed to death. They told me there was little hope for me and that I probably only had a few more months to live, no matter what was done. The cancer had spread everywhere and the tumors had wrapped themselves around some of the main blood vessels. I was understandably upset at this news but I did not lose all hope. A friend of mine had been cured of terminal cancer in Germany and I decided to go to the same doctor. I got the earliest appointment available and when the doctor examined me he said he thought my cancer was caused by the extremely toxic condition of my body. He had all my fillings replaced with nontoxic materials, gave me some homeopathic remedies and said that my cancer should be entirely gone in three to four months. Ten years have passed since that time and I have enjoyed excellent health. I feel there is no danger that my cancer will ever return, as long as I exercise regularly and keep my body reasonably clean and avoid unhealthy processed foods.

No Metal Is Safe

In the past, if a person was not found to be allergic to metals or other substances—when electro-diagnosis or muscle-testing were used—it was assumed that the material tested was not harmful. However, recently two interesting discoveries have been made which have shown that this method of testing can be misleading. Firstly, it has been found that if a small sample of a metal or other material appears to cause no allergic reaction, this does not mean that a larger amount is harmless. Secondly, it has been discovered that even if the metal some jewelry is made of causes no allergic reaction, pieces of jewelry can cause serious interference with the meridian energy flow. This applies especially to items of jewelry which surround a body part—i.e., rings, bracelets or necklaces. This is because if an acupuncture meridian is surrounded by a metal ring of any kind this always affects the energy flow. The degree of interference seems to depend on the size of the piece of jewelry. For instance, a small ring will usually cause less trouble than a heavy bracelet. This is why many leading holistic doctors recommend that their patients, especially the more seriously sick ones, stop wearing all jewelry—even if it is made of gold or other precious metals.

The following testimonials are good examples of the harmful effects that even precious metals can have if too large an amount is used.

1. "I suffered with pain in my right wrist and hand for over ten years. At times the pain was so acute that I could not use my hand at all. On several occasions I could not sign a check because I could not hold a pen in my hand firmly enough to write. Although I enjoyed playing tennis I had to give up the game because of the pain I experienced each time I tried to hit a ball. Over the years I went to many doctors seeking help, but none of them could find a reason

for my problem. Eventually, a holistic dentist—who used electro-diagnosis—said that the pain in my hand was caused by a dead tooth. He suggested that I have the tooth pulled because it was causing serious interference with the meridian energy flow. He assured me that if the tooth was removed the pain in my hand and wrist would subside. After listening to his explanation and watching him check me with the electro-diagnostic instrument, I agreed to have the tooth extracted. To my great surprise and relief soon after the tooth was gone the pain which I had for so long ceased. For five years I did not have a bridge made—to fill the gap left by the missing tooth —and I noticed that my teeth began to shift. My dentist told me that a bridge should be put in before the teeth shifted any more. For a week or so after the new bridge was installed I felt no ill effects and I was happy to be able to chew better again. My dentist had carefully checked all the materials the new bridge was made of with his electro-diagnostic instrument to make certain they caused no allergic reaction. You can imagine my surprise when about ten days after the bridge had been installed I noticed the old pain in my hand was back, worse than ever. At first I could not understand what had happened and I did not even suspect that the new bridge could be the cause. However, when the pain did not go away, but kept getting worse, I went back to my dentist. This time, when he checked the new bridge, to his surprise he found that I was strongly allergic to it. After checking further with the electro-diagnostic instrument my dentist removed the bridge—and once again the pain in my hand stopped. Further testing led to the discovery that although I showed no sensitivity to small amounts of the gold the bridge was made of, I was strongly allergic to the large amount which had to be used for the bridge. This large metal object (the bridge) in my mouth was also presumably blocking off the energy flow to my right hand and causing the severe pain."

2. "Two years ago, for no reason that I could think of, I developed serious health problems. I became weak and depressed and began having daily migraines. I was also covered in sores and welts which caused me continual discomfort. This deterioration continued and I became bedridden. Several doctors examined me and I was sent for tests, but nobody was able to find the reason for my problems. Then suddenly it occurred to me that my problems could be caused by a bridge which had been inserted not long before my sickness started. It covered five teeth and I could not think of any other major change which had taken place recently. My sister, who was now living with me, urged me to go to my dentist and have the new bridge checked with electro-diagnosis. The dentist was surprised when we contacted him and said that he had checked all the materials he used very carefully and had found that

I was not sensitive to any of them. However, he agreed to check the bridge when he heard how sick I was. To the general amazement of both the dentist and all of us, I was now found to be strongly allergic to the large bridge. When this was removed my problems soon cleared up and within two weeks I was back to normal. Further testing showed that although I showed no sensitivity to small samples of the metal the bridge was made of, I was violently allergic to the whole bridge. Presumably, my body could tolerate small amounts of the gold alloy but larger amounts had a very adverse effect.

NOTE: Gum disease is mainly caused by a lack of calcium, vitamin C, bioflavinoids, and rutin, and not just poor dental hygiene. Electro-diagnosis and muscle-testing have shown that persons with gum disease— weak, tender, inflamed, bleeding gums, pyorrhea, or loose teeth — are always low on the above nutrients. If you take enough bone meal or dolomite, which are good sources of calcium, and a supplement containing vitamin C, bioflavinoids, and rutin, you can prevent periodontal (gum) disease. If you already have it, it will soon clear up—unless it has progressed too far. You should also gently brush your gums with a soft brush as well as flossing between your teeth. You should take about 4000 mgs of vitamin C and 500 mgs of rutin daily.

CAUTION: Occasionally, people have a chronic deficiency of rutin, which is the most important deficiency in gum disease, because of a sensitivity to the materials which have been used in dental restorations—amalgam, nickel, gold, etc. In cases like this the nutritional supplements will have little effect.

5 Intestinal Parasites And Fungi

The ineffectiveness of modern methods for detecting intestinal parasites—worms, candida, Giardia—is one of the most important reasons for our failure to cope with cancer. Unfortunately, the commonly used medical procedures for discovering the presence of intestinal parasites are so inaccurate they often do more to deceive the doctor than to help him. As a result, the medical profession has been misled into believing that parasitic infestations are rare and play an insignificant part in causing sickness.

It is only since electro-diagnosis and muscle-testing have begun to be used that the enormity of the problem posed by intestinal parasites has been clearly understood. Electro-diagnosis and muscle-testing are not only more accurate than standard medical tests, they are easier to use. It is no longer necessary to spend several days waiting for the results of lab tests. With electro-diagnosis and muscle-testing it is possible to tell in a matter of seconds whether a person has parasites or not. Since these new methods of diagnosis have begun to be used, it has been found that close to ninety percent of persons tested show signs of parasitic infestation. In the case of cancer patients the fig-ure is even higher. Cancer patients practically always show signs of heavy parasitic infestation, as well as the so-called open ileo-cecal valve syndrome. This is not surprising when one considers that cancer is only a symptom of extreme toxicity. Intestinal parasites and an open ileo-cecal valve cause the body to be subjected to a continuous flood of poisons. In no other way can such quantities of toxins enter the human organism.

The ileo-cecal valve syndrome is probably the most important problem which can be caused by parasites. The ileo-cecal valve (see illustration) is located at the end of the small intestine. Its function is to prevent back flow of the highly toxic fecal matter from the colon. If this happens, a veritable river of poison pours into the body.

Until a few years ago, no one suspected that the ileo-cecal valve could malfunction and become unable to close fully in many people. The only evidence we had that the ileo-cecal valve does not function normally in some people was the evidence gathered from barium studies performed in the case of patients with intestinal problems. On the X-rays of these patients, it could sometimes be seen that the barium had not been stopped by the valve and had penetrated deep into the small intestine. However, the number of patients examined this way was very small. There was no easy, quick way of checking large numbers of people. Therefore, there was no reason to suspect that a malfunctioning ileo-cecal valve could be a common problem. Since muscle-testing has been used, it has been possible to show that in close to half the patients tested the valve does not function normally and remains open all the time. This can be a very serious problem and it can often be one of the main causes of many common conditions—such as back pain, headaches, skin conditions or fatigue. In the case of cancer patients a much higher proportion are found to have an open ileo-cecal valve. Not surprisingly, persons who have been diagnosed as having cancer show evidence of an open ileo-cecal valve practically every time.

The Alimentary Canal

This short description of the alimentary canal, or gastrointestinal tract, is included so the reader might have a better understanding of the function and importance of the ileo-cecal valve. After mastication (chewing) food passes down the esophagus (or gullet) into the stomach. Comparatively little digestion takes place in the stomach. The main function of this organ is to act as a storage tank from which the food is slowly emptied into the small intestine. It is in the small intestine that most digestion takes place. Here the food is acted upon by the pancreatic enzymes and enzymes secreted by tiny glands in the walls of the small intestine itself. These enzymes break the food down into its basic chemical components, which then diffuse through the walls of the small intestine directly into the blood stream.

The total length of the small intestine is about twenty feet. It is divided into three sections, the last of which is called the ilium. The ileo-cecal valve is located at the end of the ilium, at the point where the small intestine empties into the colon. The first part of the colon is called the cecum, hence the name ileo-cecal valve.

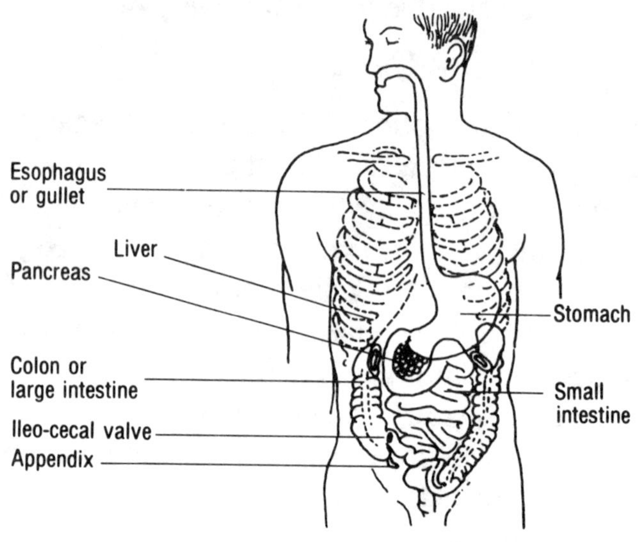

This diagram shows the different component parts of the gastrointestinal tract.

When a certain quantity of fully digested food accumulates in the end of the ilium, the valve relaxes and the food is pushed into the cecum. As soon as the food has passed through, the valve closes firmly behind it. This way the fermenting, putrefying fecal matter in the colon is prevented from backing up into the ilium.

The walls of the colon, or large intestine, are designed in such a remarkable manner that they are impermeable to the poisons inside the colon. Under normal conditions, the only way that these poisons could pass into the blood stream would be if they could somehow get back into the ilium. But this is impossible since the ileo-cecal valve remains closed and does not allow any backup from the colon into the small intestine.

Possible Causes Of An Open Ileo-cecal Valve

The reasons why the ileo-cecal valve remains open in some people are not clear and we shall probably never understand exactly what happens. There is no doubt that one of the causes is an energy imbalance. This must be so since the valve can readily be made to function normally again if the energy imbalance is corrected by touching or rubbing the acupuncture points shown at the end of this chapter. Exactly how this acupressure treatment corrects the imbalance of energy and causes the ileo-cecal valve to function normally is a mystery, as is the question of how the Chinese discovered what should be done. However, it can be easily demonstrated that immediately following the acupressure treatment, the valve always closes and begins to function normally again. As is usual with acupuncture techniques the result is always positive. If this were not so, the Chinese doctors could never have guaranteed their patients' health the way they did.

Another possibility is that if a person has parasites they, somehow, cause the ileo-cecal valve to stay open. How worms can cause the valve to remain open is difficult to understand. Nevertheless, it has been found that almost every person who has an open ileo-cecal valve also shows signs of slight irritation, or inflammation, of the entire abdomen. This irritation is thought to be caused by parasites, since it soon disappears when patients take herbs to kill parasites. Also, even if the acupressure treatment for closing the valve is not used, the ileo-cecal valve will always close once the parasites are gone.

How Common Are Parasites?

Most people are not aware of the danger posed to their health by intestinal parasites. Since lab tests are practically always negative, no matter how severely infested a patient may be, medical doctors seldom mention intestinal parasites. We also rarely see anything in the press concerning health problems caused by parasites. However, if you look in the right places you will find plenty of literature showing that a small minority of specialists are very much aware of the prevalence of parasitic infestation. For instance, in a pamphlet put out by a medical manufacturer in Phoenix, Arizona, we read:

> Colon therapy has an anthelmintic action—this means that parasites are removed. We find that over 90 percent of the people we examine in our clinics have some form of parasites. The most common of all are tapeworms. Our skilled technicians report seeing green, brown, grey, yellow and white ones—

and various combinations. Patients report seeing pieces of tapeworm in the toilet bowl, varying in length from a few inches to several feet. The longest one reported was 57 feet. Various other parasites are seen including hookworms, pinworms, whipworms, and many other exotic forms. Tapeworms are usually beef, pork or fish variety. Many vegetarians also have various parasites. Their eggs may be ingested with vegetables or fruit. Threadworms and hookworms may pass through the unbroken skin, they are sometimes picked up when one walks through the grass.

In a full-page advertisement, with a large photo of a small girl handing a pencil to a classmate, for a vermifuge called Combantrin we read in a New Zealand monthly:

The simple act of passing a pencil, sharing a book, touching the same doorknob, or even sharing a house with untreated adults is all that is required for parasites to spread—no matter how clean your child may be and no matter how careful you are. The symptoms caused by parasites may include: loss of appetite, anal and vulval itching and scratching, disturbed sleep, bloating, occasional bed wetting in younger children, swelling of the face and lymph nodes of the neck, a green or yellowish discharge in the urine, loose bowels, etc. These may seem like common occurrence in childhood, but, unfortunately, this is because the parasite problem is a common one.

I once told a patient that I thought her daily migraines were caused by parasites and an open ileo-cecal valve. I asked her whether she found this very surprising and whether she was aware that parasites are very common and often cause headaches, fatigue and other symptoms. She answered that she was aware of this since recently she had taken her children to a doctor in Germany because they were complaining of indigestion and restlessness. After examining the children, the doctor told her he found they had pinworms and these parasites were causing their symptoms. At the time she could not believe this. She told the doctor it was impossible for her children to have parasites since she insisted on the highest standard of hygiene. Also, she had not seen any signs of worms in the children's clothes or beds. But the doctor insisted and told her that over 90 percent of people in that area had parasites, so she should not feel embarrassed in any way about her children also having them. When I heard this, I no longer felt bad about telling the lady I thought she had worms. This proved to be the correct diagnosis because when she took the herbs her headaches soon improved. Yet this patient had been to a number of doctors and none of them had been able to do anything for her.

In an interview recorded in a health publication, Dr. William Kelley, the famous cancer specialist says:

I find parasites in 92 percent of people. Everybody, rich and poor, the whole population has parasites. They are not restricted to the lower classes at all. Pets are great carriers of parasites. Also, vegetables may carry parasitic organisms. One day I had a lady who was a little over 5 feet tall and weighed 300 pounds. She was on a 400-500 calorie diet and starving to death. I said, "You've got so many worms, all you assimilate is the water." This horrified her. Most people are upset at the thought of having worms. She started a bottle of special supplements I gave her but nothing happened. So she went to her family doctor who took a stool culture but could find nothing.

The lady decided to finish the bottle of supplements by taking them regularly. One night she was lying in her bed when she felt a tickling in her throat and thought it was mucous. She went to the bathroom and coughed it up, put it on a kleenex, turned the light on, looked at it and screamed, scaring her husband to death. They found the head and two more inches of a tapeworm which had come up in the throat. Lots of times, in children particularly, the tapeworm will come through the nose looking for some more to eat.

Parasites mimic a lot of diseases. Like heart trouble. I found this once. I had a nurse as a patient who had suffered with all kinds of heart trouble and went to doctors for years. She had these heart spells.

I said, "You should have gone to a vet."

She said, "Why is that?"

"Because we have found what is wrong with you, you have heart worms."

We put her on a nutritional program and she has had no more trouble since. Most stomachaches and colitis could have a parasitic involvement. Liver damage and liver trouble can be caused by worms. Sometimes a colony of worms will crawl up in the gall bladder and cause you trouble. This can be the problem with many overweight people. The worms are well fed, but the body is only getting the water and the calories and a fraction of the nutrients.

Maurice Mességué, the famous French herbalist writes this about garlic.

Nowadays statistics indicate that those parts of the world where garlic is eaten in quantity have a low incidence of cancer. Wherever I found garlic in use I found health.

From this statement we see that in areas where people eat a lot of garlic, which is the best herb for killing parasites, few have worms and an open ileo-cecal valve. As a result, the incidence of cancer is also reduced.

Diarrhea

Diarrhea is the result of an inflamed condition of the colon. In more extreme cases this condition is called colitis. If ulceration is present the name ulcerative colitis is used. Since this condition can usually be easily corrected by de-worming the patient, some experts have suggested that it is always caused by intestinal parasites. Since all patients with colon cancer have been found to be heavily infested with parasites, it has also been suggested that parasites are probably the only cause of colon cancer.

Prostate Trouble

Apart from causing difficulty in urination in some cases, inflammation of the prostate gland in men can cause lower back pain, shoulder pain, and other symptoms. Prostate trouble responds so well to large doses of garlic and other herbs which kill parasites, that it appears that in the majority of cases inflammation and swelling of the prostate are caused entirely by parasites. As in the case of colitis, all patients with prostate cancer have been found to be heavily infested with intestinal parasites. Therefore, it has been suggested that parasites are probably the only cause of prostate cancer.

How To Correct The Open Ileo-cecal Valve

This can be done in a matter of seconds by:

1. Rubbing the first point on the spleen meridian (Spleen 1). This point is located on the inside of the large toe, next to the toe nail. (See drawing below.) This must be done on both feet.

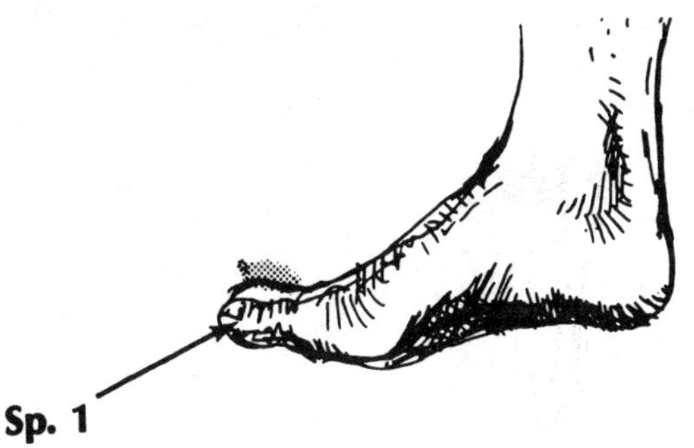

2. Rubbing the third point on the large intestine meridian. This point is located just below the knuckle of the index finger. This must be done on both hands.

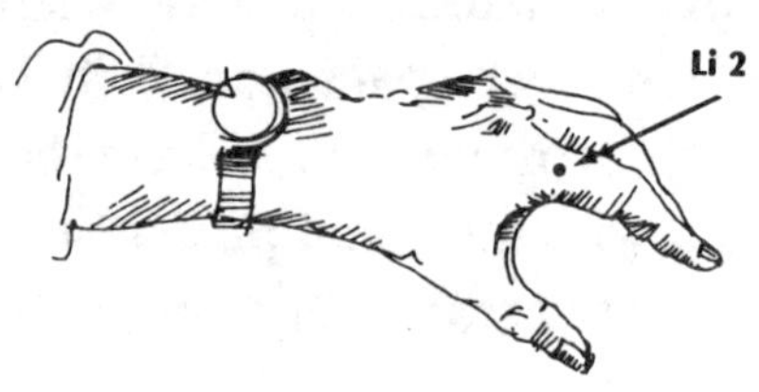

3. Touching (not rubbing) the 58th point on the bladder meridians on both legs at the same time. The point bladder 58 is located on the side of the leg, about two-thirds of the way down from the knee to the ankle. (See drawing below.) You must hold your hands straight down the sides of your calves. Fingers together and not separated. The tips of your fingers should be about two inches above your ankles.

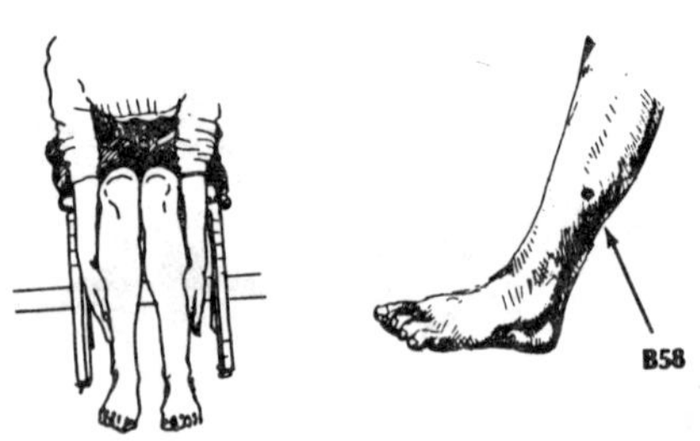

4. Touching (not rubbing) the point bladder 58 on the LEFT leg and at the same time touching (not rubbing) the point Kidney 7 on the RIGHT leg. The point Kidney 7 is located behind and below the ankle.

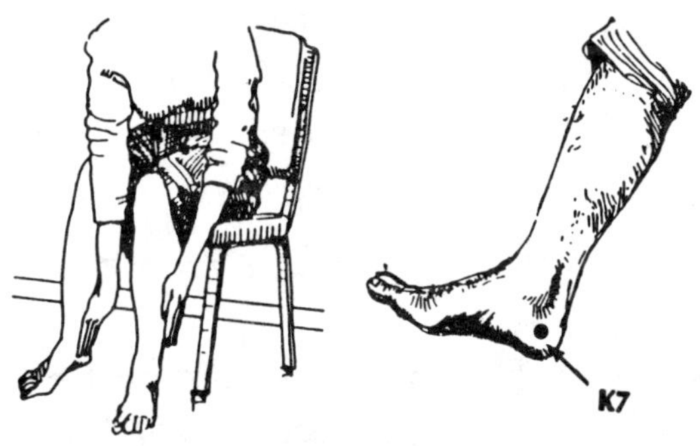

The above procedure can be carried out either by the patient himself or by another person. As is usual with acupuncture, the result is always the same. Every time the above mentioned points are treated, the open ileo-cecal valve corrects itself instantly. This shows that if acupuncture points are used correctly the treatment cannot fail to produce the desired result. If this were not so the Chinese doctors could not have been as successful as they were.

How To Rid Yourself Of Intestinal Parasites

Parasites are so common that reinfestation is certain unless a vermifuge is taken on a regular basis. Drugs are effective but may eventually cause side effects if taken too often. Herbs cause no such problems. The best are garlic, black walnut, and herbal combinations containing pumpkin seeds. However, large doses have to be taken if satisfactory results are to be obtained. If less than four or five capsules are taken at the same time, there may be no effect. The garlic and black walnut should be taken together, four or five capsules of each. The herbal combination containing pumpkin can be taken alone, but also at least four capsules at a time. The best time to take these herbal capsules is just before dinner.

Homeopathic remedies can also be used effectively to kill parasites. They are especially useful for persons who cannot take herbs. Special preparations consisting of defatted almond flour, fig powder and other ingredients are also available for small children and infants.

The above remedies should be taken daily for the first month or so, and after that once or twice a week to ensure that the parasites do not return. Candida can best be treated with homeopathic remedies.

Fungi

Fungi, or yeasts, are believed to form part of the normal intestinal flora. The most common of these yeasts is candida albicans, or candida for short. We hear more about candida than any of the other yeasts because it is believed to cause the most trouble.

Since yeasts are so common, and they are found in everyone's digestive tract, how do we know that they are harmful? When they were first discovered it was believed that yeasts played a useful part in digestion and it was not suspected they could cause problems. When it became common knowledge that many symptoms can be alleviated by reducing the intake of refined carbohydrates (sugar, white flour, etc.) it was suggested that this happened partly because refined carbohydrates cause yeasts to proliferate excessively. This belief was strengthened even more when drugs, the best known of these is nystatin, began to be used to control yeasts. The use of these drugs often produces such marked improvements that many symptoms are now believed to be caused by yeasts. The list is endless, ranging from fatigue, headaches and back pain to arthritis and various infections.

As a result of these findings it is now believed that as long as the immune system is strong, the body can prevent a yeast overgrowth. The yeasts remain in the digestive tract and not only do no harm but are believed to be useful in helping digestion and assimilation. If the body becomes rundown and weak the yeasts may proliferate excessively and invade other parts of the body. This happens most readily if refined carbohydrates are overindulged in. Refined carbohydrates are bad for the body and weaken it, while they promote rapid growth of the yeasts.

An interesting discovery has also been made concerning the possible relationship of fungi to cancer. When homeopathic remedies, which kill a far wider spectrum of yeasts than drugs, began to be used for controlling fungi it was found that it is not unusual for so-called cancerous tumors to disappear when these homeopathic remedies are taken regularly. Presumably, fungal growths can be easily misdiagnosed as being cancerous tumors.

6   Misalignments of the Skeleton

Another important reason why no satisfactory solution to the cancer epidemic has been found is that misalignments of the skeleton have been entirely disregarded by researchers. Medical doctors are taught nothing about these misalignments and their harmful effects. Only osteopaths and chiropractors try to help their patients by adjusting the spine and extremities.

The most scientific research to discover the effect of spinal misalignments has been that conducted by Dr. Ralph Gregory in Monroe, Michigan. Dr. Gregory soon noticed that the spinal misalignment which causes the greatest problems is that of the atlas vertebra. This is the spinal bone the head rests on. Because the atlas is so close to the brain, even the slightest misalignment of this important vertebra plays havoc with normal body function.

Dr. Gregory's research has shown that when the atlas vertebra misaligns, and begins to interfere with nerve impulses passing along the spinal cord, the muscles on one side of the back immediately spasm and can no longer relax normally. This involuntary contraction of the back muscles twists and distorts the spine as shown in Fig. #1.

If the atlas vertebra can be realigned so the pressure on the brain stem is relieved, the back muscles relax and the body straightens out, as shown in Fig. #2.

Precision X-rays and postural checks developed by Dr. Gregory have shown that virtually everyone's atlas vertebra is misaligned and is pressing on the brain stem. As a result, everyone's body is twisted by the spasming muscles.

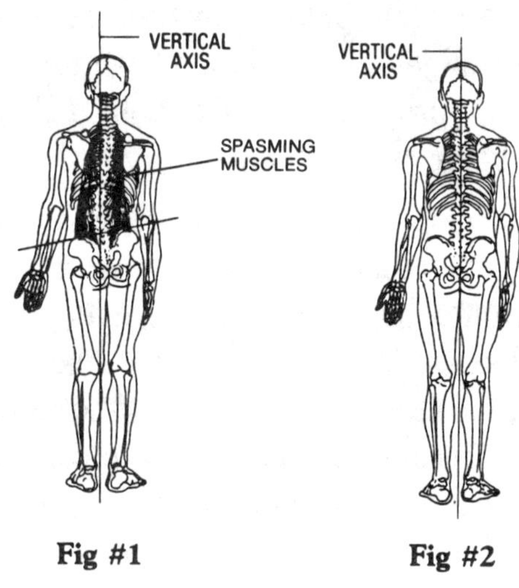

Fig #1   Fig #2

Fig. #1 This illustration shows the effects the atlas misalignment has on the spine and pelvis. It can be seen that the atlas has moved to the left. This has caused spasming of the muscles of the right side of the back. As a result, the spine is bent sideways (this is known as scoliosis) and the pelvis is tilted.

Fig. #2 If you compare this illustration with Fig. #1 you can see the change in the alignment of the entire body which takes place when the atlas is adjusted. When the pressure is removed from the brain stem, the muscles of the back relax and the spine and pelvis straighten out.

The misalignment of the atlas vertebra causes the following problems:

1. Interference with the normal functioning of the nervous system.

2. Nutritional deficiencies and abnormal changes in body chemistry.

3. Osteo-arthritis, or degenerative arthritis, of the spine.

4. Scoliosis of the spine.

5. Lowered hormone levels.

6. Uneven development of the muscles of the back and pelvis.

7. So called "fixations" of the spine.

These problems exhaust the body and interfere with normal function. They weaken the immune system and increase our chance of developing cancer and other degenerative diseases. Not surprisingly, there have been a number of well documented cases of terminal cancer patients who recovered spontaneously after their atlas vertebra was adjusted. When the pressure on the brain stem was removed, they became so much stronger and healthier they were able to fight off the cancer.

Interference With The Nervous System

A misaligned atlas vertebra interferes with the nervous system in two ways. Firstly, by compressing the nerve tracts in the brain stem it prevents nerve impulses, both to and from all parts of the body, from reaching their destination. Secondly, the spasming back muscles and twisted vertebrae press on the spinal cord and spinal nerves, shutting off normal nerve supply to many parts of the body.

The symptoms which result from the misalignment of the atlas vertebra may, therefore, vary enormously. Pain, weakness, or malfunction can occur in any part of the body. The atlas misalignment plays an important part in causing headaches, back pain, fatigue, dizziness, numbness, sciatica, pain radiating down the arms, malfunction of organs, and practically every known health problem.

Nutritional Deficiencies And Abnormal Changes In Body Chemistry

The constant spasming of the muscles on one side of the back drains the body of energy and exhausts its supplies of necessary nutrients. Electro-diagnosis and muscle-testing have shown that people whose atlas vertebra is misaligned invariably have far more and greater deficiencies of vitamins and minerals. Those persons whose muscles can relax normally, because their atlas has been aligned, show far fewer deficiencies.

The most important deficiencies caused by the atlas misalignment are those of calcium, trace minerals, and vitamin E. Electro-diagnosis and muscle testing have shown that persons whose atlas is misaligned are low in these important nutrients practically all the time.

Calcium

The calcium deficiency, associated with the atlas misalignment, is due to the spasming muscle using up far more calcium than would normally be the case. As a result, a calcium deficiency is found even in persons who take calcium supplements regularly and eat foods which are high in this essential mineral. The atlas misalignment plays an important part in causing such common problems as tooth decay, osteoporosis in older people, muscle cramps, pain and stiffness of the neck and shoulder muscles, chest pains, shortness of breath and other symptoms associated with a lack of calcium in the organism.

Trace minerals

Another important nutritional deficiency which is always found in persons whose atlas vertebra is misaligned is that of trace minerals. A lack of trace minerals can cause a host of problems such as headaches, dry skin, poor assimilation, brittle hair and nails, fatigue, lack of stamina, etc.

Vitamin E

Amazingly, electro-diagnosis and muscle-testing have shown that persons whose atlas is misaligned are always lacking in vitamin E, while those whose atlas vertebra has been aligned are never low in this essential vitamin.

When the atlas vertebra is aligned, and the body can finally relax normally, the deficiencies of calcium, trace minerals and vitamin E soon cease. Patients often experience remarkable improvements in health if their atlas is kept aligned for a period of several months or years. Sometimes, significant relief of symptoms is felt much sooner.

Osteo-Arthritis Or Denegerative Arthritis Of The Spine

Osteo-arthritis of the spine is the name given to the degenerative changes which take place in the spine as we get older. It is also referred to as degenerative arthritis.

Osteo-arthritis of the spine plays an important part in causing most of the health problems of older people. On an average, it shortens their life by at least ten years. Those persons whose atlas vertebra remains aligned do not develop osteo-arthritis of the spine, especially if they keep the muscles of the back strong with special exercises. Osteo-arthritis of the spine is more fully discussed in the next chapter.

Scoliosis Of The Spine

When the muscles on one side of the back spasm uncontrollably as a result of the pressure on the brain stem by a misaligned atlas vertebra, the spine will curve to one side (see Figure #1). If the curvature becomes very pronounced it is known as scoliosis of the spine. This condition can easily be corrected if the atlas vertebra is adjusted in time and a program of special exercises is followed. Since spinal curvatures of this kind cause extremely uneven stress on the vertebrae and the spinal joints, degenerative changes are likely to develop rapidly. When these changes become too extensive the curvature may become impossible to correct fully.

Lowered Hormone Levels

Over fifty years ago Dr. William Sutherland, a doctor of osteopathy, discovered that all the bones of the skull move rhythmically as we breathe. This movement is essential for the normal functioning of the brain and the flow of the cerebrospinal fluid, the fluid in which the brain and spinal cord are suspended. Therefore, if the bones of the skull misalign and stop moving normally, this can cause serious interference and chronic problems.

One of the largest and most important bones of the skull is the sphenoid. This bone forms the anterior part of the floor of the cranial vault. The pituitary gland, the master gland whose hormones control the function of many important glands of the body, is located in a small groove in the upper surface of the sphenoid bone. The rhythmic movement of the sphenoid with respiration is essential for normal functioning of the pituitary gland.

Electro-diagnosis and muscle-testing have shown that the deficiency of trace minerals, which invariably develops when the atlas vertebra misaligns, interferes with the normal movement of the sphenoid and this in turn interferes with normal pituitary gland function. When this happens, hormone levels drop significantly and many important body functions slow down. When the atlas vertebra is aligned and the trace mineral deficiencies disappear, the sphenoid soon begins moving normally again and hormone levels improve.

Common Problems Caused by Hormone deficiencies

The most important deficiency which results from the misalignment of the sphenoid is that of estrogen. Therefore, indirectly, the atlas misalignment can cause such problems as irregular menstrual periods, infertility, menstrual cramps, and a chronic calcium deficiency. Estrogen, a hormone produced by both sexes, is essential for normal calcium utilization. When levels of estrogen drop, calcium can no longer be adequately metabolized. As already mentioned, this can result in cavities, osteoporosis, muscle weakness, and a host of other symptoms related to a lack of calcium in the organism. The misalignment of the sphenoid bone is also the main cause of headaches.

Uneven Muscle Development

The tilting of the pelvis and the general twisting of the skeleton, caused by the atlas misalignment, result in uneven development of the muscles of the back and pelvis. If the muscles on one side of the body become a lot stronger than the corresponding muscles on the other side, the pressure on the spinal cord and spinal nerves may become so extreme that very serious health problems can develop. Placing the patient on a program of unilateral exercises is the only way to correct this form of muscle imbalance. When the muscle imbalance is corrected, truly amazing results can sometimes be obtained. Disabling health problems, for which no solution could previously be found, may gradually correct themselves.

Fixations Of The Spine

If the muscles in certain parts of the back spasm very severely, the corresponding sections of the spine will become rigid and stiff. The parts of the spine where normal mobility is lost are known as "spinal fixations." When the atlas vertebra is aligned, the muscles of the back relax and spinal fixations disappear. The back exercises shown in the next chapter are also very helpful in relaxing the muscles of the back and restoring normal mobility.

Adjusting The Atlas Vertebra

The most consistent and successful method for correcting misalignments of the atlas vertebra is that developed by Dr. Ralph Gregory. This scientific, precision adjusting technique is sometimes referred to as the N.U.C.C.A. method. Dr. Gregory is the founder and president of N.U.C.C.A., the National Upper Cervical Chiropractic Association.

So many hopelessly sick patients with every kind of problem have been helped when their atlas vertebra was adjusted, that people have travelled from all parts of the world to be treated by Dr. Gregory.

Some Case Histories

The following five case histories have been included to give the reader a more graphic understanding of the problems which may arise as a result of the atlas becoming misaligned because of an accident, a blow, or some other mishap.

1. Following an auto accident this young woman experienced severe migraine headaches, nausea, dizziness, and back pains. Even the strongest pain killers gave little or no relief. Chiropractic manipulation of the spine did help significantly, but there was no long term relief and sometimes the patient had to be taken to the doctor as many as three times a day. She had to spend over six months in bed in a darkened room, unable to open her eyes most of the time.

When this patient came to have her atlas vertebra adjusted she was carried into the office dressed in her robe and pajamas. She was semiconscious and never said a word. Following the adjustment of the atlas there was no improvement, but the next day the patient came back fully recovered. She had no further problems.

2. This fifty-six-year-old patient experienced progressive loss of strength and coordination in his legs. He went to numerous specialists and spent well over thirty thousand dollars on tests and various treatments. But no doctor could find anything wrong and the treatments did not help. The gradual deterioration continued.

When this patient's atlas was adjusted no immediate improvement was noticed. In fact, the following day he was much worse. He improved steadily after that and regained the strength and coordination in his legs.

3. An elderly female patient experienced such severe neck and shoulder pains when she woke up one morning that she had to be taken to a hospital by ambulance. Extensive tests and examinations were all negative, but the pain

did not diminish in spite of the administration of morphine every four hours. After a month of treatment with drugs, traction and physical therapy there was no improvement. The patient was steadily getting worse and threatened suicide.

When this patient's atlas vertebra was adjusted her pain immediately stopped and never returned.

4. Following an auto accident this thirty-five-year-old patient experienced severe headaches, neck and shoulder pain, weakness, nausea and numbness of the arms and shoulders. She spent four months in bed. She was examined by several specialists but no reason could be found for her problems. She gained over thirty pounds and became very weak, something that distressed her greatly since she was a good tennis player and loved to exercise. When this patient's atlas vertebra was adjusted all her problems immediately ceased.

5. For forty years this middle-aged man had suffered with frequent migraines and severe dizziness, to the point that he often lost his balance and fell. He consulted many specialists but no reason could be found for his problems. He was treated by medical doctors, osteopaths, chiropractors, etc., but there was no change in his condition. When this patient's atlas was adjusted, using the N.U.C.C.A. precision method, all his problems cleared up. He has not misaligned again and has had no further trouble. He had only one treatment.

SUMMARY

The atlas misalignment causes such severe interference with normal function that no treatment can be fully successful unless the atlas is also realigned. Adjusting this important vertebra should be the first step in any successful preventative health program. Virtually everyone's atlas is misaligned and most headaches, back pains, and other health problems are largely a result of this misalignment.

The N.U.C.C.A. precision adjustment is so gentle that the patient feels nothing when his atlas is being aligned. Dr. Gregory found that by reducing the force of the adjustment a far greater degree of accuracy can be achieved.

By disregarding misalignments of the atlas vertebra, Western medicine has overlooked one of the most important causes of chronic health problems.

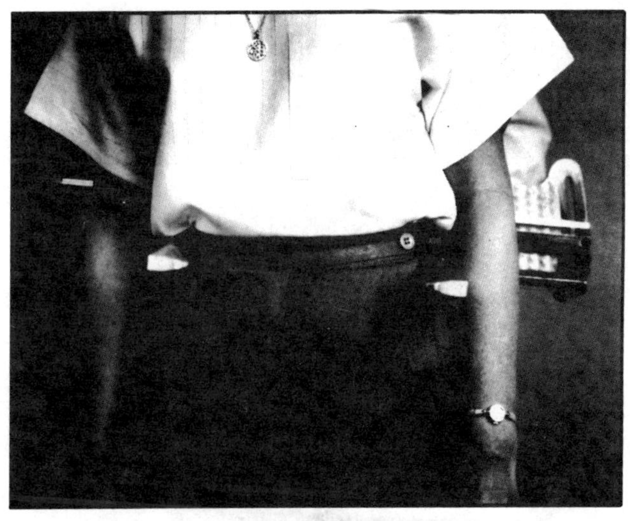

Fig #3 This photo shows a patient being checked for misalignments on the Anatometer. This scientific, precision instrument was designed by Dr. Gregory. It is the most accurate instrument ever made for detecting and measuring postural abnormalities. The measuring arms of the Anatometer are placed firmly on the patients pelvic bones and locked in position. The patient is then asked to step off so that pelvic tilt and rotation can be recorded (see photo on next page).

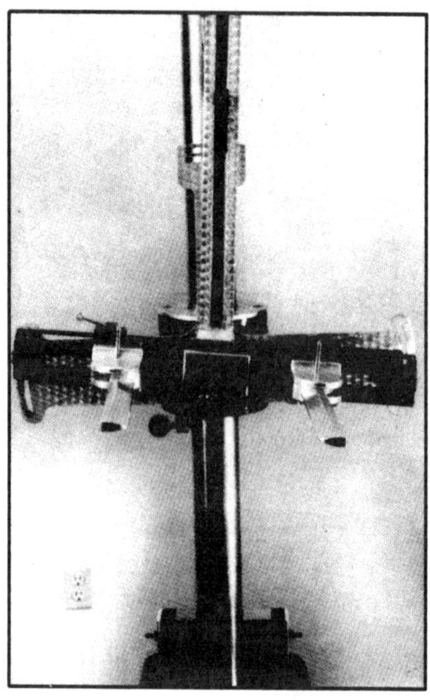

Fig # 4 This photo shows the Anatometer after the patient stepped off. The tilt of the measuring arms shows the degree of misalignment of the pelvis. Since the Anatometer has begun to be used it has been found that practically everyone has a badly misaligned pelvis and hips. This could not be accurately determined before since there were no precision instruments for this purpose.

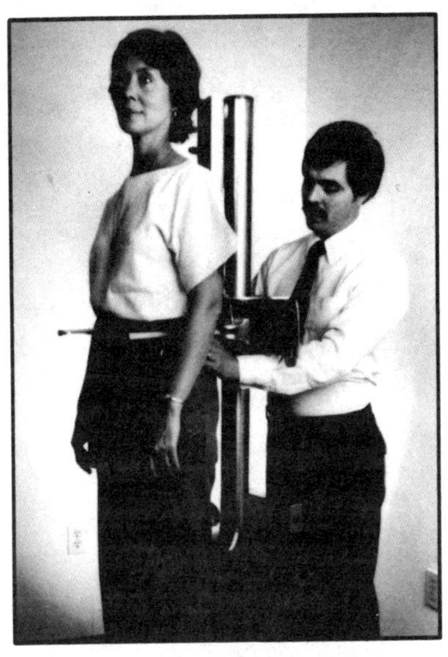

Fig #5 In this photo the patient is being checked on the Anatometer after her atlas was adjusted using the scientific, precision, N.U.C.C.A. adjusting technique. Her hips are now level since the spinal muscles have relaxed and they have allowed the spine and pelvis to realign themselves.

Patients who have had their atlas adjusted by using other methods seldom show a complete relaxation of the back muscles. When checked on the anatometer their hips are still found to be uneven. Although manipulation of the spine can produce loud "cracks" and "pops", which give the illusion that the spine has been adjusted, it cannot be used successfully for adjusting the atlas. The anatometer has shown that after manipulation, the spasm of the back muscles never improves. Sometimes it may even become worse.

The End Of Cancer

7 Osteo-Arthritis Of The Spine

If cancer is an unfortunate medical blunder, then osteo-arthritis of the spine is an even greater blunder. While cancer affects only a quarter of the population, osteo-arthritis of the spine affects practically everybody over the age of thirty-five. This form of arthritis plays an important part in causing virtually every health problem of older people. It shortens the average person's life by at least ten years.

The reason why osteo-arthritis of the spine has received so little attention is because doctors have not understood its causes. They have wrongly assumed that it is an inevitable consequence of the aging process. As a result, organized medicine's treatment programs for this kind of arthritis are in most cases limited to dispensing pills. No attempt is made to prevent the condition.

Osteo-arthritis, or degenerative arthritis of the spine, is the name given to the degenerative changes which take place in the spine as we get older. (See illustrations.) These changes most often begin during middle age, but in individuals who participate in strenuous physical activities and sports, the spine can become seriously damaged even before the age of twenty.

The degenerative changes in osteo-arthritis consist of:
1. A wearing out and narrowing of the spinal discs.
2. Changes in the shape of the vertebrae.
3. The growth of sharp spurs on the edges of the vertebrae.
4. Eventual fusion of the vertebrae.

The chief problems caused by these degenerative changes are stiffness, pain, and extreme interference with the nervous system. This inevitably leads to a progressive lowering of resistance to disease and a loss of vitality. Osteo-arthritis of the spine is probably one of the main reasons why older people develop cancer more often.

The Causes Of Degenerative Arthritis

The spine can be compared to a very strong flexible steel rod. It is stabilized from all sides by powerful muscles and ligaments. As long as the muscles hold the vertebrae firmly in their correct position, damage to the spinal joints cannot occur. The spinal joints can become damaged only if they are subjected to abnormal stress. This can happen in two ways. First, as already explained in the previous chapter, when the atlas vertebra misaligns and presses on the brain stem all the muscles on one side of the back will spasm. This involuntary contraction of the back muscles results in constant uneven stress on the spinal joints. Sooner or later degenerative changes in the spine will inevitably develop.

Secondly, as also mentioned in the previous chapter, uneven pressure on the spinal joints occurs if the muscles of the back become unevenly developed. If this happens the vertebrae twist and it is only a matter of time before the spinal joints begin to show signs of wear. The most serious damage occurs if the muscles which stabilize the spine from behind become weaker than those in front of the spine. If this happens the spine loses its flexibility and the spinal discs degenerate rapidly. (See illustrations.)

Symptoms Caused By Osteo-arthritis Of The Spine

These symptoms can be divided into two groups—those caused by interference with the nervous system and those which result from the stiffness and pain which accompany degeneration of the spine. Common symptoms caused by pressure on the spinal cord and the spinal nerves are: weakness, numbness, tingling, shaking, angina pains, etc. Most frequently affected are the arms, shoulders and neck, but all parts of the body may be involved. The chronic pain and stiffness, which result from degeneration of the spine, make exercise difficult and cause increasing weakness and debility.

Prevention Of Osteo-arthritis Of The Spine

Since this form of arthritis consists entirely of mechanical damage and is not due to physiological changes and calcium deposits, it is one of the easiest conditions to prevent. All you have to do is keep your back muscles strong with regular exercises and make certain your atlas vertebra remains properly aligned. As long as your back muscles are strong and hold the vertebrae firmly in place, your spine cannot degenerate.

Americans are, generally speaking, a "quick fix" oriented nation. We are always looking for a drug, a pill, or some gadget which will control the problem. As a result, medical research has degenerated into a continual search for "magic cures." Simple, inexpensive, common sense solutions are disregarded, especially if they require some personal effort and self-discipline. Nowhere is this more true than in the cases of cancer and osteo-arthritis of the spine. Billions of dollars of tax monies, have been wasted in the hopeless search for "quick fixes." Common sense tells us that no gimmick will ever be found which can solve the problem of cancer or of degeneration of the spine.

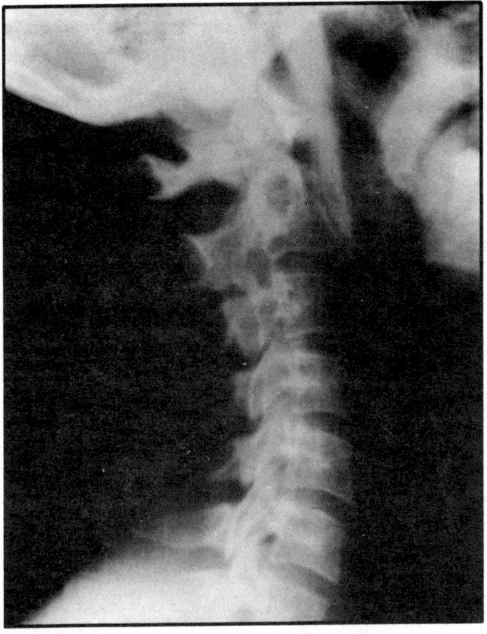

Before looking at X-rays of spines which show arthritic changes, let us examine the X-ray of a healthy spine.

The cervical (neck) spine shown in this X-ray is as near perfect as possible. The discs are all thick and healthy, of uniform thickness and not narrower at the back and wider in front. The bodies of the vertebrae are all uniform in shape and almost the same size. The forward, or lordotic, curve is excellent. Notice how uniform it is. This indicates that the spinal muscles are strong.

Unfortunately, only a very small minority have good necks like this, and well over 90% have weak necks which show a loss of the normal curves.

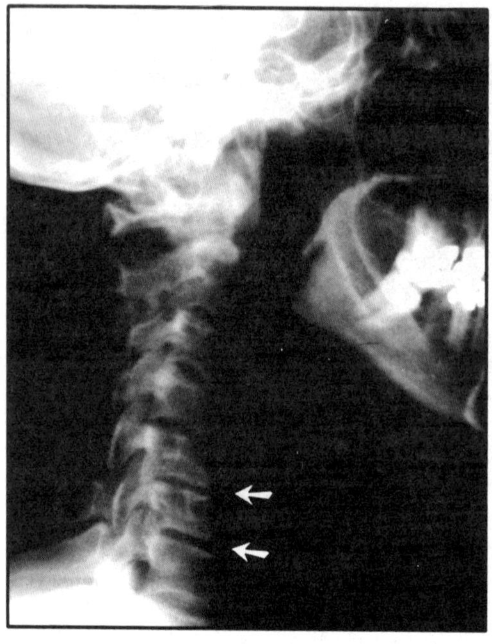

This patient's neck shows a reversal of the normal cervical curve due to weakness of the muscles of the neck. Because of this the joints of the lower neck are seriously damaged.

This patient's left arm was so weak that she could not raise it to shoulder level. But after six months of exercises to strengthen her neck muscles and home traction using a towel, the muscles of her left arm and shoulder recovered their normal strength— since the pressure was removed from the spinal nerves. The patient was 51 years old at the time the X-ray was taken.

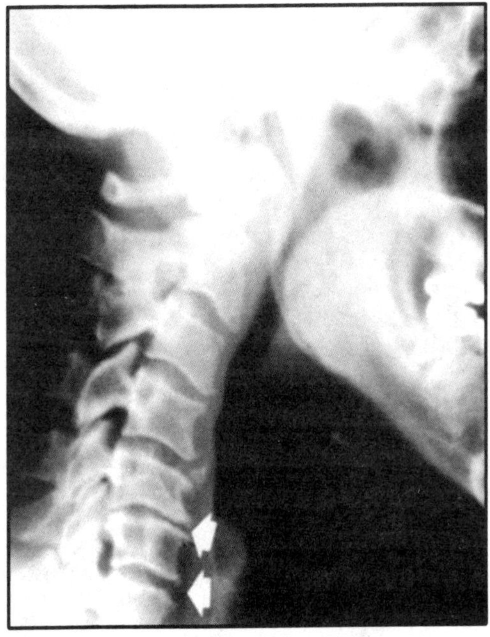

This patient's neck shows a reversal of the normal cervical curve due to weakness of the neck muscles. As in all such cases, the spine is seriously damaged. The patient complained of daily migraines, but these stopped immediately when he was adjusted and started doing exercises to strengthen his neck muscles. In this patient's case cervical traction using a rolled up towel was especially helpful. The patient was 55 years old at the time the X-ray was taken.

When the osteo-arthritic spurs press on the spinal nerves, this pressure can result in quite unexpected symptoms. Cervical traction, using a rolled up towel, has proved effective in cases of angina pectoris, shooting pains in the neck, shoulders and chest, numbness, tingling, etc.

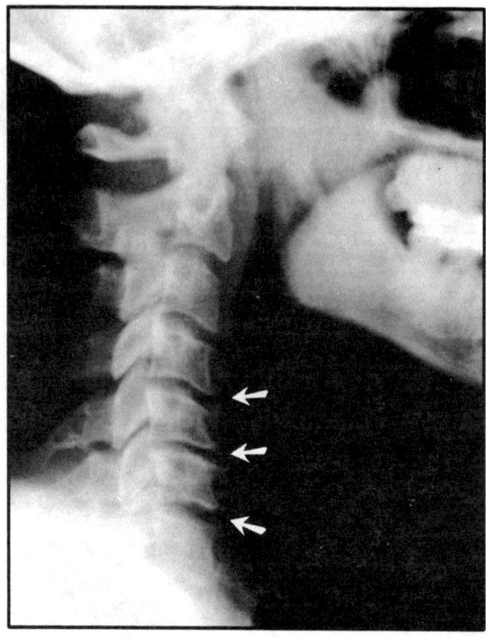

You do not have to be elderly to have a degenerated spine. This patient was only 36, and he shows all the classic signs of degenerative arthritis; spurring, flattening and widening of the bodies of the vertebrae, and thinning of the discs. He was a very athletic individual and enjoyed such sports as skiing, tennis, etc. If you engage in a lot of physical activity when you are misaligned and have a weak back, then you are likely to ruin your spine at an early age.

Contrary to what one would expect, athletes often have the worst spines and their cervical spines are often curved the wrong way. This is because most exercise programs are badly designed and develop the spinal muscles, and other muscles, unevenly.

Spinal Exercises For The Prevention Of Degenerative Arthritis

Weakness of the muscles which hold the vertebrae in place is the main cause of so-called osteo-arthritis, or degenerative arthritis of the spine. This can be such a health-destroying, debilitating condition that every possible effort should be made to prevent its onset.

Regular exercises to strengthen the spinal muscles are our best guarantee against osteo-arthritis of the spine. As long as the back muscles are strong and hold the vertebrae firmly in place, it is impossible for this form of arthritis to gain a foothold. But once it is allowed to start and nothing is done to check it, it will spread like a cancer throughout the spine, destroying the discs and the spinal joints and eventually making normal function and health an impossibility.

Prevention of osteo-arthritis is one good reason why regular exercises to strengthen the back muscles are important. Prevention of spinal misalignments is the other. If the spinal muscles are strong, they can easily prevent the vertebrae from misaligning and pressing on the spinal nerves and the spinal cord.

When the vertebrae are not held firmly by the muscles, they soon start slipping out of place. They then press on the spinal nerves and interfere with the normal transmission of nerve impulses to various parts of the body. This pressure on the nerves results in such problems as weakness, pain, malfunctioning of organs, numbness or headaches.

Should Everyone Do The Spinal Exercises?

Yes! Even if you are very fit and already do a lot of exercise, you should still include back exercises in your program. In fact, athletes often have a greater need to do these exercises than persons who do little exercise. This is because the main problem is not so much weakness of the spinal muscles as uneven development of these muscles. The back muscles of persons who do a lot of exercise are often far more unevenly developed than those of individuals who exercise little.

If the back muscles become unevenly developed, the stronger muscles twist the spine in their direction. The normal curves are lost and the spine becomes vulnerable to injury and degenerative changes. Unless something is done to correct this, damage to the spinal joints and discs will develop automatically.

The main purpose of the exercises, therefore, is not just to strengthen the back muscles, but to strengthen them as evenly as possible, producing a well balanced spine which will never deteriorate.

When your spinal muscles are well balanced, your spine will regain its normal curves and the vertebrae will be held firmly in exactly the correct position. You will be surprised how much better you will feel. Your head will be clear, you will have more energy, and your entire body will function better because there will be no pressure on the nervous system. The flow of nerve impulses from the brain to all parts of the body will be restored to normal and may be better than ever before in your life.

You should always remember that the spinal muscles are designed in such a marvelous way that when they are strong and well balanced, the vertebrae will be held in exactly the correct position at all times—when you are sitting, standing, running, carrying some heavy weight or twisting in any direction. This in itself shows that Nature attaches great importance to preventing pressure on any part of the nervous system, which is the master control system of the body.

Before starting any exercise program you should always make certain that your atlas is aligned, and is not causing your body to be twisted. If your entire body is misaligned, as a result of an atlas misalignment, exercise will tend to cause muscular imbalances to become worse.

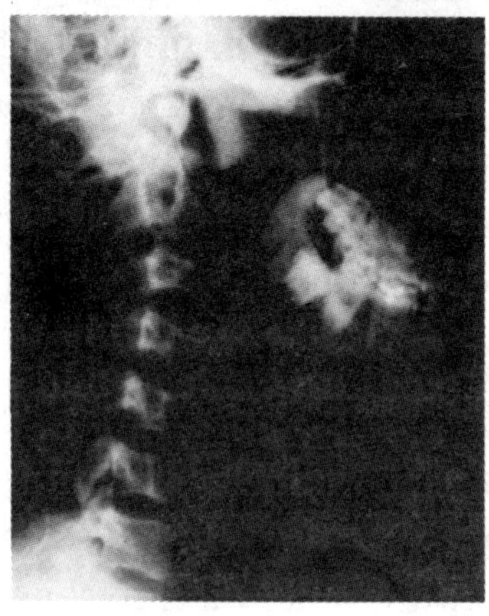

Illustration #1—This photograph shows an X-ray of the cervical (neck) spine. The two main symptoms of weakness of the spinal muscles can be clearly seen. A loss of the normal forward (lordotic) cervical curve and irregularity. By irregularity we mean that the vertebrae are not well lined up and show a staggered or stair stepping effect. The line formed by the backs of the bodies of the vertebrae is called George's line. It forms the anterior or front wall of the neural canal through which the spinal cord passes. If the vertebrae are badly misaligned because of weakness of the spinal muscles, as is the case in this illustration, there will be pressure on the spinal cord and the spinal nerves, with consequent interference with the normal flow of nerve impulses to some parts of the body. A neck like this is weak and the spinal joints will wear out causing osteo-arthritis to set in at an early age.

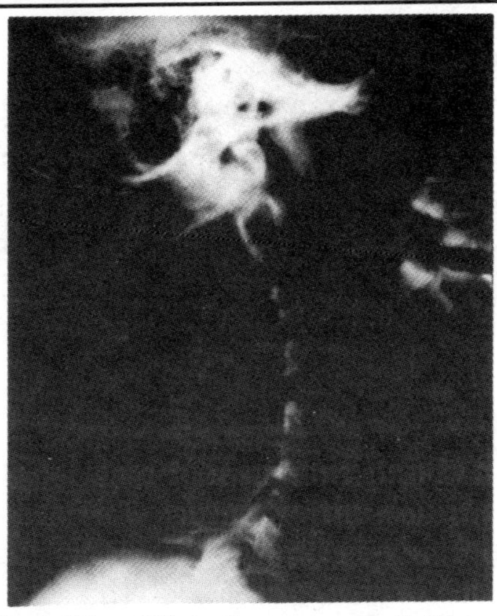

Illustration #2—This is a second X-ray of the same patient whose cervical X-ray was shown in illustration #1. This X-ray was taken 21 days later, after a program of exercises to strengthen the spinal muscles. It can be seen that once the spinal muscles became strong, they automatically pulled the vertebrae back into their correct positions and aligned the spine perfectly. The backs of the bodies of the vertebrae now form a smooth line and there is no pressure on either the spinal cord or the spinal nerves. As long as the spinal muscles remain strong and hold the vertebrae in perfect alignment, degenerative arthritis, or osteo-arthritis, can never set in. Notice the perfect forward curve.

Everyone can have a spine like this if he does the exercises regularly and makes certain he remains in good adjustment by going for a checkup two to three times a year. School children should be taught the exercises at an early age. It is easy to develop a good spine while one is still young. The later one starts the harder it becomes.

Spinal Exercises

These exercises strengthen and stretch the spine and make it both strong and flexible. The vertebrae will then be held firmly in place and will not press on the nervous system. The formation of fixations can also be prevented as explained later in this chapter. However, you should be careful not to overdo these exercises when starting. Too much too soon can be harmful.

Whenever doing exercises keep the following rules in mind:

1. Increase slowly as you feel yourself getting stronger.
2. Never do too much. Only do that which you can handle easily.

If you overdo, you will get stiff and sore; you might even pull a muscle or strain ligaments which may be very painful. This could discourage you and stop you from continuing with the program.

It should be kept in mind that all exercises will not strengthen the spine. Frequently, yoga teachers and athletes have very weak spines and loss of the normal spinal curves. To have a strong spine and good spinal curves you must do *exercises specifically designed* to strengthen the spinal muscles. Just being fit is not *enough*.

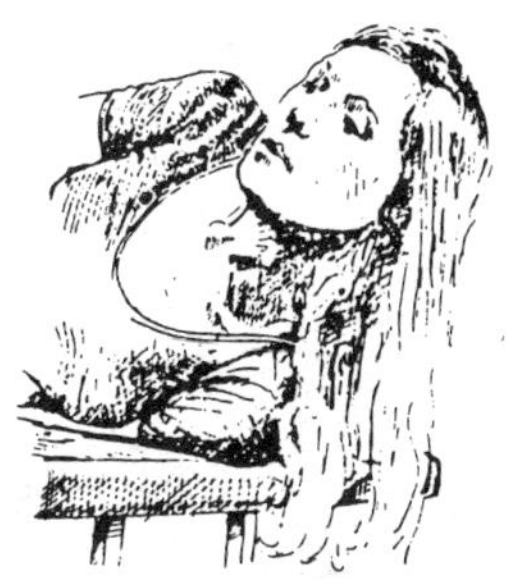

Exercise #1

For this exercise you must lie on your side with your head over the edge of a bed or bench. Lower your head as far as you can and then lift it as high as you can. This should be repeated 30-40 times. The best time to do the exercises is in the morning before rising. If you do them in bed, you will find that this will loosen and warm you up so you will be much better prepared to start the day.

Exercise #2

Lie on your back with your head over the side of your bed or a bench. Drop your head as low as you can, then raise the head as high as you can. Repeat 10-20 times.

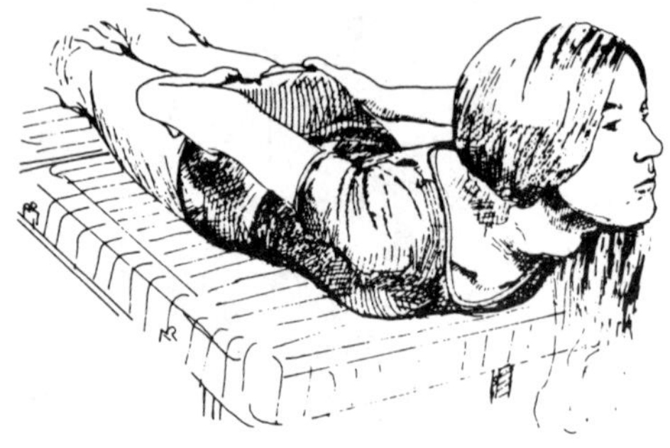

Exercise #3
For this exercise, lie on a bed on your stomach, with your head and shoulders over the edge. Lower your head as far as you can; then lift the head and upper torso as high as you can. *Do not move your legs.*

At first you can repeat this exercise only a few times, but as you become stronger you should try to increase to a hundred or more repetitions. This is by far the best exercise for strengthening the muscle at the back of the neck. These muscles are especially important in holding the vertebrae in place. They are more important in this respect than the muscles at the sides or front of the spine. Do the repetitions fairly quickly. If you do them slowly the exercise will take too long and you will be tempted to give up.

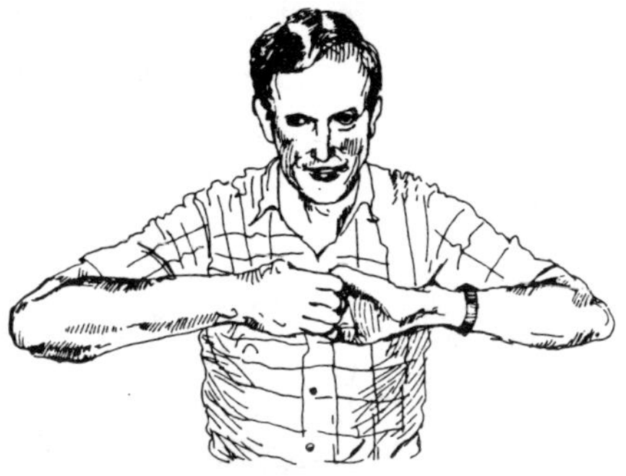

Exercise #4
Clasp your hands firmly in front of you and pull apart to the count of 4 or 5. Relax for a few seconds and repeat 5 to 10 times. This exercise can be done several times a day. Lying on one's back in bed or while sitting or standing. It is the best exercise for strengthening the muscles of the upper back and shoulders. If you do this exercise several times a day and strengthen the muscles of the upper back sufficiently, you will never have pain in this area unless you become very deficient in vitamins, trace minerals or manganese.

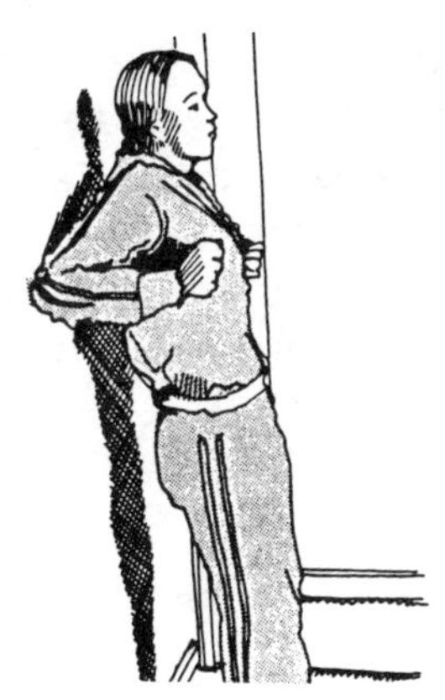

Exercise #5
Stand with your back to the wall and push yourself away with your elbows. Do this 20-40 times. As you get stronger, place your feet further and further away from the wall.

This is another excellent exercise for strengthening the upper back and shoulders.

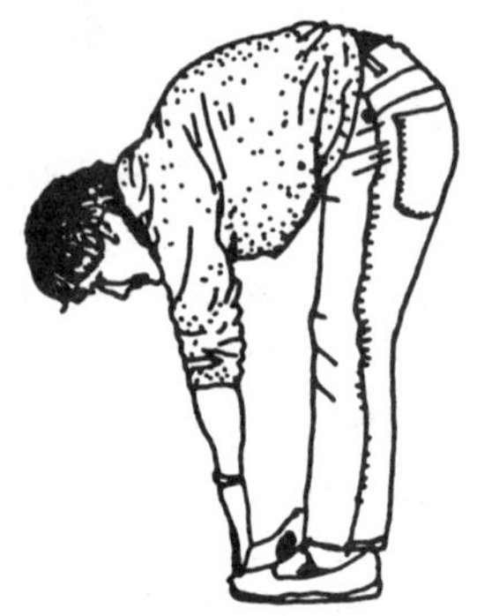

Exercise #6
Unless something is done to prevent it, the muscles in your lower back, as well as your hamstrings, will gradually shorten and become stiff. This may result in the development of "fixations" in the lower back, discomfort and even lower back pain. The only ways to prevent shortening and stiffness of the above muscles is to include the exercise shown in this drawing in your daily exercise program. Before trying to touch your toes make certain that you are warmed up. If your muscles are stiff and cold you may injure them and give yourself a backache.

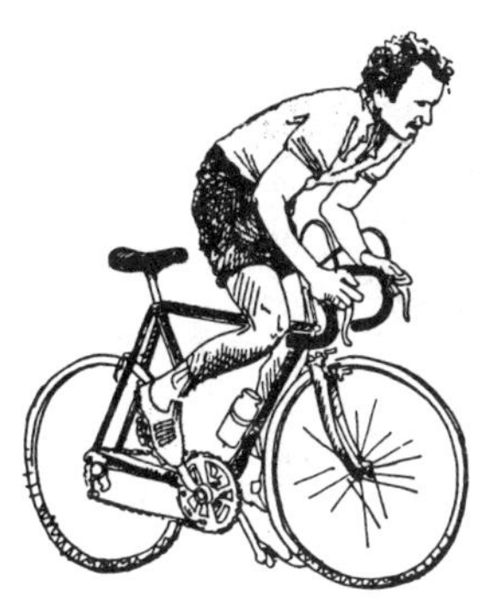

Exercise #7
Riding a bicycle is probably the best exercise for strengthening the muscles of the lower back and pelvis. Make a habit of going for an hour's ride as often as possible; especially if you have already had lower back trouble and your back muscles are weak. Riding a bicycle up a gradient is especially good.

Exercise #8
The purpose of this exercise is to stretch the muscles and ligaments of the pelvis (especially the psoas muscle). Make sure your heel does not come off the surface of the chair, and the leg that you extend behind you remains as straight as possible. Maintain this position for 10 to 15 seconds.

This exercise is especially helpful in cases of back trouble or scoliosis. It should be repeated two to three times a day.

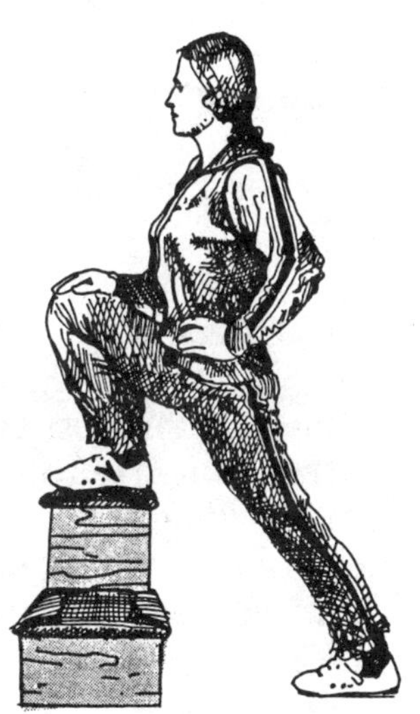

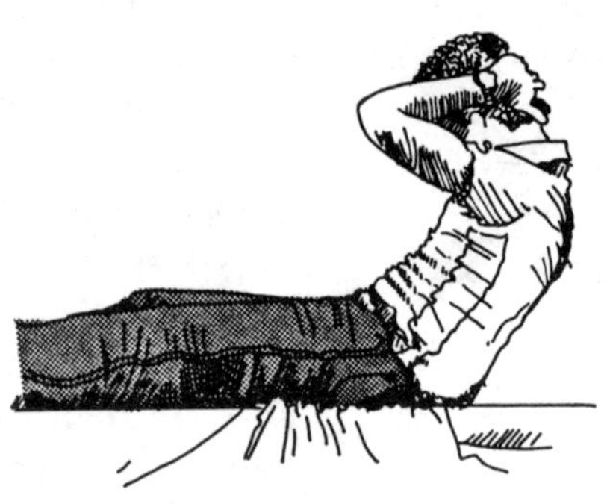

Exercise #9
When doing sit-ups do not start by trying to do a large number with your hands behind your head, as shown in the drawing above. You should start by doing just one or two and increase gradually. If you are having a lot of difficulty at first, try putting a thick pillow, or even two pillows, under your back to make it easier for you to start with.

If you find doing sit-ups too difficult, you can try raising your legs. At first raise the legs one at a time. When you can raise each leg five to ten times, then try and raise both legs at the same time. Strengthening the stomach muscles will not only help prevent back trouble, but strong abdominal muscles also help hold the organs in place.

It has been known for a long time that weakness of the stomach muscles is an important cause of

back trouble. The stomach muscles counterbalance the pull of the back muscles. Consequently, if the stomach muscles are weak the back muscles may pull the spine out of shape causing a condition known as "sway back." Here the lower back curves forward excessively. This frequently occurs in persons who are overweight and exercise very little.

Exercises to Strengthen the Arches

One of the important discoveries about the body made by using muscle testing is that if a person has weak arches this can seriously weaken the back, especially the lower back.

Wearing arch supports is an easy way of solving the problem of weak arches, but only partly. This problem can never be fully corrected unless daily exercises to strengthen the arches are used.

The best exercises to strengthen the arches are walking on the toes, riding a bicycle pressing on the pedals with the ball of the foot, or doing so-called toe raises.

The easiest of these exercises is walking on the toes. This can be done at any time during the day without having to take time off from other activities. If toe raises are to be effective, you should do them three or four times a day, forty or fifty at a time. This, however, is time consuming and hard to keep up. Walking on the toes is by far the easiest and most practical. If you walk on your toes enough each day, within two or three months your arches will be strong and they will no longer trouble you.

Weak arches are not restricted to only those persons who have flat feet. Muscle-testing shows that most people have weak arches to some extent. This is probably so because we walk on hard surfaces most of the time and we also wear stiff, hard soled shoes most of the time. Even if you think that you have good arches you should make a point of walking on your toes and doing toe raises as often as possible.

Spinal Traction

Because of the upright position that we are forced to remain in for most of the day, our spines have to become compressed to some extent. The only way to overcome this is by different forms of traction. This can often produce wonderful results.

The most effective way to stretch the neck at home, without any expensive equipment, is by rolling up a towel and placing it under the neck with the head hanging over the edge of the bed or couch, as shown in the diagram. The towel should be folded, as shown, so that there is a soft spot in the middle once the towel has been rolled up. The neck will fit into this soft spot. As the towel is placed under the neck it will tend to bend the neck forward restoring the forward lordotic curve. Since the head is hanging over the edge, the weight of the head will pull on the neck and this will exert a certain amount of traction on the cervical spine. For this form of traction to be effective you have to lie, with the towel under your neck, for at least 12 minutes. You should do this at least three to four times a week, but preferably every day.

How to Fold the Towel

The towel must first be folded in two, then folded in two again. When folding it the second time you fold it from both sides so that the two ends do not quite meet, leaving a gap of about half an inch. Now you roll the towel up as tightly as you can to produce a firm roll. The roll will have a soft middle because of the gap that was left when folding the towel. This soft middle part is for the neck to fit into. Now the rolled up towel is placed on the edge of a bed or bench and you can lie down with your head over the edge and your neck on the roll. Place another roll under your low back. Lying like this will help to restore the normal curves to the spine.

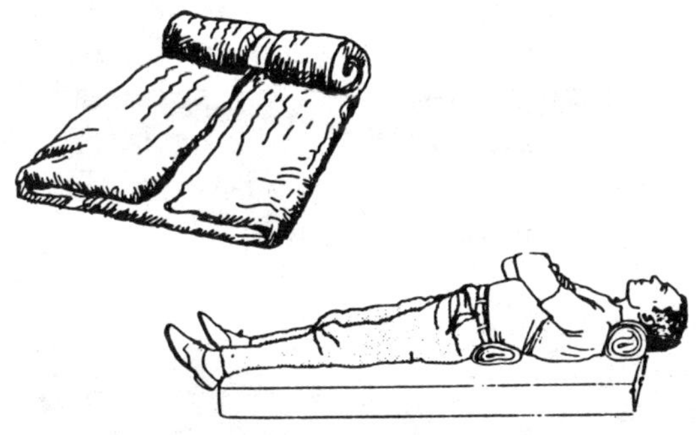

Roll up a towel as shown in the diagram above. Place the towel under your neck on the edge of a bed or couch so that your head is hanging over the edge. This is an excellent form of home traction for the neck and will sometimes stop headaches almost at once, because the neck muscles relax. To prevent the neck from getting stiff, turn your head very slowly from left to right every 40-50 seconds or so.

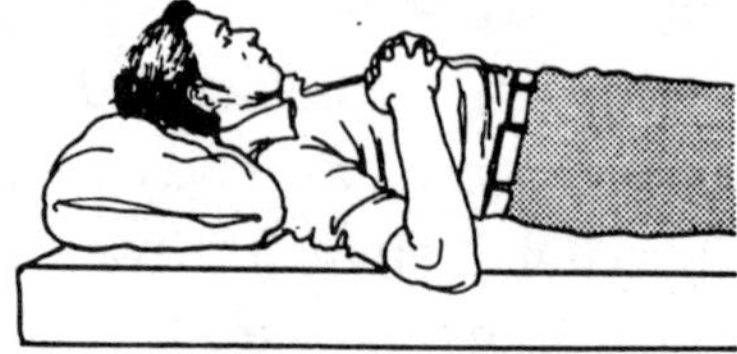

When X-raying people's necks, one finds that about 90% or even more have bad necks with some or all of the normal curve lost and replaced by a straight neck. Quite often the cervical spine is actually bent backwards. The reasons for this are not clear, yet it is likely that the main reason is sleeping on a pillow which supports the head but does not support the neck, as shown in the above drawing. If you remain in this position for the whole night, your cervical spine is bound to lose its normal curve sooner or later. Nobody should use a regular pillow. The only pillow which is good is an orthopedic pillow.

This is a drawing of an orthopedic pillow without the pillow case on it. It shows the high edges and low trough in the middle. The high edges support the 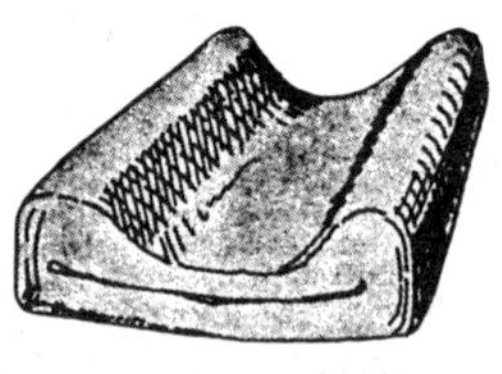 neck while the head rests in the trough. This is the only kind of pillow to use. The neck is the most important part of the body when you are sleeping and it should be correctly supported.

Fixations

As mentioned in the previous chapter, important enemies of the spine and of normal function are so-called "fixations." If the spine is under constant stress because of a misaligned pelvis, the muscles which hold the vertebrae in place cannot relax as they normally would. They continually try to pull the misaligned vertebrae back into their correct positions. These muscles may become so tense that they will go into spasm causing the joints in that part of the spine to become locked or "fixed".

In the part of the spine which has become "fixed", motion is either reduced considerably or there may be no motion at all. Most of these "fixed" areas are quite painless. However, in certain cases the muscles in the area of the fixation may become acutely painful, causing severe backache and disability. In fact, spasm, an involuntary persistent muscular contraction, seems to be one of the most important causes of back pain.

How Fixations Can Be Relaxed

As mentioned above, the main cause of fixations is misalignment of the pelvis. This always results in misalignment of the entire spine and causes some of the spinal muscles to become stiff and tense as they vainly try to realign the back. As previously explained, the pelvis is pulled out of alignment because some of the major muscles which stabilize it become weak. When the body is balanced (by adjusting the atlas) these weak muscles will regain their strength and realign the pelvis. Once the pelvis is aligned again, relaxation is noticed throughout the back, and some or all of the fixations disappear at once or in a few days. If a backache is solely due to spasming muscles around "fixed" parts of the spine, the backache may stop either immediately or in a day or two, depending on the degree of muscle spasming.

The second most important cause of "fixations" is simply stiffness of the spine due to lack of exercise. If you do very little or no spinal exercises or, for that matter, no exercises of any kind, but instead spend hours over a desk, typewriter or sink, then your spine is bound to get stiff and fixations may develop even if you are in good adjustment. Therefore, once the spine has been adjusted, the best way of removing the remaining fixations is to do the back exercises regularly to strengthen and stretch the spine.

8　Preventing Cancer

Since cancer is nothing more than a symptom of an extremely toxic condition of the body and a breakdown of the immune system, it is one of the easiest health problems to prevent. This is especially true as cancer does not develop quickly. It often takes as long as twenty years before the toxic load becomes so great that tumors begin to appear. Therefore, you usually have lots of time to decide when you want to start on your program of cancer prevention.

To prevent cancer all you have to do is keep your body functioning reasonably well and prevent excessive accumulations of toxins in the tissues. The best and easiest place to start is your diet. You can start cleaning up your eating habits right away.

The Macrobiotic Diet

The macrobiotic approach has been used successfully in saving large numbers of cancer patients who had been given up as hopeless by orthodox medicine. The main purpose of the macrobiotic method is to cleanse the body and strengthen the immune system. One of the best books on the prevention of cancer with the use of macrobiotics is "The Cancer Prevention Diet," by Michio Kushi. In this book the author, who has treated thousands of cancer patients successfully, writes:

As long as we continue to take in excessive nutrients, chemicals, and other factors which serve no purpose, they must accumulate somewhere in the body. If we don't allow them to accumulate in limited areas and form tumors, they will spread throughout the body and cause a total collapse of our vital functions and death by toxemia. Cancer is only the terminal stage of a long process. Cancer is the body's healthy attempt to isolate toxins ingested and accumulated through years of eating the modern unnatural diet and living in an artificial environment. Cancer is the body's last drastic effort to prolong life, even for a few more months or years. By gathering the unwanted materials in local areas, the rest of the body is maintained in a relatively clean and functioning condition. This process of localization is part of our natural healing power, saving us from total breakdown. But the modern view looks on those localizations as dangerous enemies to be destroyed and removed. Its attitude can be compared to the behavior of the inhabitants of a city troubled with too much waste. Instead of investigating the source of the waste, the city dwellers blame the sanitation department for the accumulated garbage, in designated locations, and decide to do away with the sanitation department.

Cancer is not the result of some alien factor over which we have no control. Rather it is simply the product of our daily behavior, including our thinking, life-style, and daily way of eating. We must go beyond looking at cancer at the cellular level and realize that our cells are constantly changing in quality, being nourished and rejuvenated as a result of nourishment and energy coming into them. Whatever is in the nucleus of a cell is nothing but the end result of what originally came in from the outside and formed the cell components. If the cell is abnormal, something coming in is abnormal, such as the blood, lymph, or vibrational energy including electromagnetic waves from the environment.

The cell is only the terminal of a long organic process and cannot be isolated from its surroundings and other body functions. Instead of focusing on the cell, we need to change the blood, lymph and environmental conditions that have created malignant cells. Instead of treating isolated organs in the body, we need to treat the source of nourishment and other factors going into those organs and change the character of those organs. The proper place to perform cancer surgery is not in the operating room after the disease has run its course, but in the kitchen and in other areas of daily living before it has developed. By removing certain foods from the pantry and refrigerator, replacing them with the proper quality and variety of foods, and applying proper cooking methods, together with correcting environmental conditions and our daily way of life, we can ensure that cancer and other degenerative illness do not arise.

The standard macrobiotic diet consists of approximately fifty percent whole grain cereals, twenty-five percent vegetables, and five to ten percent beans and sea vegetables, and five percent soups. There are a number of excellent books on the subject of macrobiotics. The names of some of them are given at the end of the introduction. It is strongly recommended that you read these books and make a careful study of this new dietary approach to preventing cancer and other degenerative conditions.

Compatible Foods

Compatible foods are those which can be digested at the same time. Our digestive system is constructed in such a way that it can cope with only one type of food at a time. This means that proteins and carbohydrates cannot be digested together. Carbohydrate digestion comes to a standstill when protein digestion is taking place and vice versa. For instance, when one eats meat, the stomach secretes an enzyme called pepsin whose function is to break down proteins. Pepsin is secreted by glands in the walls of the stomach. These glands also secrete acid so that during protein digestion the contents of the stomach become highly acid. It is only in this acid medium that the enzyme pepsin can function. If, during protein digestion, the acidity in the stomach is reduced, the digestion of protein stops because the enzyme pepsin becomes deactivated in a medium which is not sufficiently acid. Therefore, if meat is eaten with some other foods which reduce the acidity in the stomach, the digestion of the meat is slowed down tremendously.

Nature obviously intended all animals to eat one food at a time. In the natural state animals never mix their foods. Their meals always consist of a single food. The only creature who eats several different kinds of food at the same meal is the human. This creates incredible digestion problems. We regularly mix proteins with carbohydrates. Since they cannot be digested together one has to wait until the other has been digested. This, of course, slows down digestion greatly and the food remains in the stomach far longer than it should. Putrefaction and fermentation are bound to take place with a consequent increase in the toxicity of the body.

If one wants to remain healthy, it is better not to mix foods at the same meal. It would be best, of course, if one could eat just one food at a time. It would not only simplify digestion, but also reduce the temptation to overeat. This is, unfortunately, impossible under modern conditions. Therefore, everyone should have some knowledge of which foods are compatible and can be eaten together at the same meal. By eating foods which digest well together you can increase your energy enormously and prevent many health complications.

Be Sure To Chew Your Food Well

Although this may not be obvious at first sight, your chances of developing cancer could depend to some degree on whether you chew your food well or not. In nature, foods cannot be swallowed without first being well masticated. Everyone knows that it is impossible to swallow nuts, apples, or almost any other natural food without chewing it first. Obviously, it is nature's plan that we chew our food well and at the same time mix it thoroughly with saliva. Not understanding the importance of proper chewing we violate this law of nature almost every time we eat. In many instances we have so changed the food Nature has prepared for us that it is virtually impossible to chew it at all. As a result, we become so used to swallowing our food without proper chewing that when we are eating something that really needs chewing, we try to swallow it before it has been properly broken down. The most critical in this respect is meat. Eating foods that require little or no chewing can make one so lazy that one is inclined to swallow meat after chewing it only slightly. If meat is well masticated it will seldom remain in the stomach for more than three or four hours. But , if meat is not well broken down, the pieces may remain in the stomach for twenty four hours or more. Obviously this will slow down digestion greatly and a lot of fermentation and putrefaction will take place. The toxic load is increased substantially. Poorly chewed vegetables and breads will cause less trouble than poorly chewed meat, but in the long run this, too, may cause a serious problem.

In summary, you should avoid soft, refined foods which cannot be chewed properly. Instead try to eat wholesome, natural foods—fruits, nuts, whole grain cereals—which cannot be swallowed without proper chewing. Train yourself to chew every mouthful between twenty or thirty times. If you can develop the habit of chewing your food well, your health is bound to improve substantially.

Allergies

Electro-diagnosis and muscle-testing have shown that contact with something one is allergic to causes immediate interference with the flow of energy in the body. It is, therefore, not surprising to find that allergies to foods and other substances can have a far more important influence on our health than most laymen are aware of. The majority of people think of sneezing, asthma or hives as being the only symptoms of allergies. It has now been found, however, that a great number of other problems can also be due to allergies. The list of symptoms in books on allergies includes such unlikely conditions as diabetes, epilepsy, headaches, ulcers, canker sores, learning disabilities, sinusitis, back pain, low blood sugar and many others.

Another unusual fact about food allergies, which many people may find interesting, is that foods to which a person is allergic may cause him to gain weight. Several researchers have reported dramatic weight loss in some of their patients when they eliminated allergic foods from their diet. The following is a quotation from the book "Don't Settle For A Migraine Headache," by Dr. George Malcom:

> Two of my patients, a musician aged 24 and a farmer aged 36, were found to have cheese sensitivity. When this single item was eliminated from their diets both lost over forty pounds and their lower back pain stopped. The same weight reduction has been seen in many of my patients.

> This surprising weight loss has led me to consider the whole question of obesity. If a person drinks

too much fluid, the body just gets rid of the excess. So if one eats too much, why doesn't the body just void it also? It would seem that the allergic foods take a hold in the body and won't let go. Dr. Coca, in his book Pulse Test, also describes weight loss by eliminating food allergens.

As mentioned above, eating a food one is allergic to causes immediate interference with the flow of energy along the acupuncture meridians. At first (that is for the first few minutes,) this is so marked that it causes a general weakness. After a while, the body presumably manages to neutralize the undesirable factors in the food and the weakness begins to decrease. It seems likely, that the energy flow does not return entirely to normal for several hours, or possibly in some cases for several days. It is not surprising, therefore, to find that truly miraculous results can often be achieved by eliminating all those foods one is allergic to from one's diet.

The following is a list of foods and other substances which electro-diagnosis and muscle-testing have shown everybody to be allergic to:
- All fruit skins with the exception of fruits with very delicate skins such as cherries, cherry tomatoes, or some grapes.
- All unripe fruit. (It is surprising that the two halves of the same apple or pear can produce different effects. The half which is ripe causes no reaction, but the half which is not ripe causes an allergic reaction.)
- Iceberg lettuce.

- Many brands of chewing gum.
- Many brands of soft drinks.
- Most tap water and some bottled waters.
- Bananas. (The reason for this is hard to understand. Perhaps the starch in this fruit is changed by storage.)
- Most brands of granola, protein powders and other powdered foods such as flour. These foods oxidize rapidly after being ground up and they soon become rancid. If fresh they are all right.
- Most oils and fats. These also soon become rancid. (If fresh, they are all right.)
- Some deodorants, cosmetics, lipsticks and hair sprays.
- Raw egg whites.
- Most homogenized or pasteurized milk and many cheeses.
- All foods containing refined sugar.
- Just about all drugs.
- Tea, coffee, alcoholic beverages and bottled or canned juices.
- Some meats, spices and dressings.
- Many dried fruits.

The following is a list of foods which seldom cause an allergic reaction when checked by using electro-diagnosis or muscle-testing:

- Almonds. (This is probably due to their comparatively low fat content which helps them stay fresh longer than other nuts.)
- Most fruits when peeled.

- Romaine lettuce.
- Cooked eggs and raw egg yolks.
- Most raw or lightly cooked vegetables.
- Honey, but only very occasionally. (Most varieties of honey produce an allergic reaction when tested.)
- Distilled water.
- Fresh, whole grain foods.
- Bread made with sour dough, not yeast. (The flour bread is made of must be freshly ground. It soon becomes rancid.)
- Raw, fresh, untreated milk and fresh butter made out of unpasteurized milk.

The rule seems to be, don't eat foods which have been damaged by man. Try to eat only those foods which are fresh and as natural as possible.

Because allergies often go undetected, it is important to make certain the foods which you and your family are eating do not cause an allergic reaction.

Testing for allergies with electro-diagnosis is very simple. All substances which cause an allergic reaction also cause interference with the normal flow of energy in the body. This interference can be easily picked up with the electronic instruments used in electro-diagnosis.

It is important to check not only foods but also cosmetics, hair sprays, skin creams, jewelry, rings, watches, toothpastes and other objects with which we come into daily contact. Substances the body is sensitive to not only interfere with the energy flow along the meridians but also cause chronic low grade inflammation of the tissues with cause chronic low grade inflammation of the tissues with which they are in contact. Number one in this respect are amalgam fillings and other toxic materials used in dentistry.

From the above it can be seen that unless allergies are taken into consideration some people may never get well, no matter what other treatment program may be followed.

Stay Fit To Stay Alive

It has been known for a long time that exercise has a profound effect on health and on the immune system. The body's vitality and resistance increase almost immediately when we exercise. In view of what is now known of the important role our immune system plays in protecting us from cancer, it is not surprising to find that statistics show that people who exercise regularly also have a lower incidence of cancer. For instance, a recent report on an eight-year study of over thirteen thousand people showed that those who exercise regularly have significantly lower death rates from cancer. This study was conducted by the Institute For Aerobics Research in Dallas and published in the Journal of the American Medical Association. The study concluded that even moderate amounts of exercise help build immunity to disease. During the study among men who exercised regularly the death rate from cancer was almost four times lower than among men who did not exercise. Among women the difference was even more significant. The incidence of cancer among women who exercised regularly was over sixteen times lower than the incidence of cancer among those women who did not exercise. The death rates from heart trouble and other ailments were also significantly lower among those men and women who exercised.

Smoking

The use of cigarettes, cigars, pipes, chewing tobacco and snuff is one of the leading causes of cancer. It accounts for over thirty percent of our cancer deaths. If you smoke you should do everything in your power to stop. If you don't smoke, don't start.

Pesticides

Electro-diagnosis has shown that virtually everyone living in civilization shows signs of pesticide poisoning to some degree. This results in abnormalities in the body chemistry and weakens the immune system. Removing traces of pesticides from the tissues is an important step in both cancer prevention and cure. Fortunately this can now be done easily with homeopathic remedies which have been specially prepared for this purpose. The Hubbard detoxifying program can also be very useful in ridding the body of unwanted chemicals and other toxic substances. A medical doctor who works at a Hubbard Detox Center told me he has seen many cases where skin cancers sloughed off by themselves when the program was completed.

Lead Poisoning

It has been known for some time that lead has a strong carcinogenic effect. It is well known that people who live near freeways, or other areas where the air contains a high percentage of lead from exhaust fumes, have a higher than average incidence of cancer. When checked with electro-diagnose many people show signs of heavy metal poisoning. These toxic metal contaminants can also be removed from the tissues with homeopathic remedies and the Hubbard detoxifying method.

Toxic Materials Used In Dentistry

As already explained in chapter four, the toxic materials used in dentistry are among the most dangerous known carcinogens. Finding a good dentist who uses electro-diagnosis is, therefore, one of the first steps in cancer prevention.

Chemicals In Our Food

It is now widely recognized that chemicals in our food—preservatives, coloring agents, taste modifiers, etc.—play an important part in causing cancer. You should try to eat fresh, organically grown foods which have not been sprayed or otherwise contaminated with dangerous chemicals. Start your own garden, join a natural foods co-op, or find a store which sells organically grown vegetables and fruits.

Rancid Fats

The fat in oils, nuts, butter and other foods is often rancid. Rancid fats are especially harmful and they are known to have a carcinogenic (cancer-producing) effect. Try to obtain fresh butter made from untreated milk. Homogenized, pasteurized milk is unhealthy and causes allergic symptoms in everyone.

Intestinal Parasites

As already explained in chapter five, intestinal parasites are so widespread that hardly anyone is entirely free of them. They are one of the most frequent causes of cancer. You should never go more than three or four days without taking herbs or homeopathic remedies which kill parasites.

Cleansing

To work most efficiently and with the least effort the body must be kept clean. A buildup of toxic waste in the tissues interferes with normal function and can eventually lead to cancer. Poor bowel elimination plays an important part in this respect. Since refined foods and a lack of exercise do not provide the necessary stimulation, most people have only one bowel movement a day, sometimes only every two or three days. In such cases, the feces may form hard crusts on the walls of the large intestine. Some experts claim that older persons often have several pounds of this hardened fecal matter adhering to the walls of their colon. You should make certain that your diet contains enough roughage to stimulate normal bowel movements. Bran is excellent for this purpose as it swells up and provides bulk. Taking psyllium and herbal formulas containing cascara sagrada also helps make you more regular. These herbs also help remove the hardened feces from the walls of the colon.

The degree to which cleansing is important in the prevention and treatment of cancer can best be seen from the case histories in Dr. Max Gerson's book "A Cancer Therapy,

Results Of Fifty Cases." One of the most important objectives of the Gerson treatment is cleansing. Well before World War II, while testifying before a Senate Sub Committee, Dr. Gerson said, "Skin cancers and beginning cancers are easy to treat."

Chelation

Most people over the age of fifty, sometimes sooner, suffer with so-called atherosclerosis or hardening of the arteries. When this condition becomes more advanced complete blockage of the blood vessels may result. Common problems associated with arterial blockage are angina pains, strokes, heart attacks, inability to think clearly, memory loss, fatigue, etc. In extreme cases blockage of the arteries which carry blood to the lower limbs and feet may cause gangrene and necessitate amputation.

Chelation is a new process now being used for removing calcium deposits and the yellowish plaques containing cholesterol found in atherosclerosis. Chelation therapy involves the intravenous injecting of chelating agents which dissolve the deposits of calcium and cholesterol in the blood vessels. The most commonly used chelating agents are EDTA (a synthetic amino acid,) vitamin C, and other amino acids.

Experts familiar with chelation now believe that this new procedure could play an important part in cancer prevention. EDTA and other chelating agents are believed to strip the protein coat from around cancer cells and make it easier for the T-lymphocytes (white blood cells whose function it is to destroy invading organisms) to kill cancer cells.

It is also known that cancer grows more easily if the oxygen supply to the cells is reduced. When chelation improves circulation and allows full oxygenation of the tissues, cancer cells probably find it harder to establish a firm foothold.

Some cancer experts believe that, on an average, cancer is often present in your body for seven years or more before it is discovered. Older persons could, therefore, benefit in two ways from chelation. Cancer cells in their bodies would be more easily destroyed and the amount of oxygen supplied to their tissues would increase.

Another great advantage of chelation is that it boosts the body's immune system tremendously. Since our immune system is our number one defense against cancer, chelation makes it easier both to prevent and destroy cancer.

As with other natural therapies, organized medicine has done everything in its power to stop the use of chelation. Many doctors who used this method were taken to court and had to put up a desperate fight to keep their professional licenses to practice. This is not because chelation is dangerous in any way but because it competes with heart surgery. Recently, however, heart surgery has come under attack, and chelation is beginning to be used by more and more doctors. Chelation therapy improves the circulation in the entire body and is relatively inexpensive, while heart surgery improves the blood flow in only a few heart vessels. It is also very expensive and can even be life threatening.

If you want to learn more about chelation you should read the books "The Chelation Answer" and "Bypassing Bypass." They are listed at the end of the introduction.

Nutritional Supplements

It is now a well established fact that vitamins and minerals play an important part in strengthening the immune system, and helping to prevent cancer and other health problems. Especially important in this respect are Vitamin A, Vitamin C and Vitamin B17, or Laetrile.

Research has also shown that vitamin and mineral deficiencies are often the main cause of pain, fatigue and other health problems. By taking vitamins, minerals, herbs and other nutritional supplements regularly it is often possible to produce tremendous improvements in health as well as relief from chronic aches and pains.

Avoid Known Cancer Producing Habits

The following are some known cancer producing practices which should be either eliminated entirely or reduced to a minimum:

Frequent drinking of very hot beverages, excessive use of salt, coffee, animal proteins and drugs, overexposure to the sun, prolonged irritation of the skin by chemicals, emotional stress, smoking, etc. All of these factors depress normal function and lower our resistance.

The Importance Of Positive Thinking

Although this subject cannot be covered adequately for lack of space, you should never lose sight of the tremendous importance of right thinking and the power of the mind to heal. It is a widely recognized fact that positive emotions—such as faith, love, forgiveness, acceptance and happiness—can influence our health immensely, as well as stimulating our immune system. Some experts even believe that cancer patients who experience unexplainable remissions of their symptoms often do so because of an improvement in their mental attitude.

Every thought we think affects the function of the nervous system, the glands, cells and every organ of the body. You will notice that the healthiest people are often those with pleasant dispositions, whose focus is toward helping others achieve happiness and fulfillment, rather than selfish care for personal gain.

Happy people do not usually give way to anger and pettiness. They use the power of their minds to maintain equilibrium. They do not harbor resentments over incidents of the past since their energy is being used in trying to make the most of the present. They are relatively free of hostility and irritability because they exercise control over negative thoughts and emotions.

In other words, you could do everything recommended in this book but if you continue to think in a negative manner, placing your attention on illness rather than on health, it could all be for naught. Negative thinking can often literally destroy all other positive actions you may take.

Health also depends on having worthwhile goals. If you stay busy, you will remain healthy. When you no longer have something to live for, your body will sense this and will stop functioning effectively. Some people do not live long after they retire because they retire not only from their jobs but also from life itself. They fail to develop new interests and new goals.

Staying healthy and trying to improve oneself in every way is, in itself, a worthwhile goal. Few of us realize our full potential. We become depressed because of our lack of strength, endurance, or mental power, not realizing that it is our duty to develop these talents. Disciplining oneself and giving careful attention to what one eats and how one exercises is not only beneficial to the body but also to the mind and spirit. One not only becomes healthier but also spiritually more fulfilled. Our body has been amazingly created and it tries to adapt to every circumstance of life. If we work at it with courage and perseverance we can develop our God-given talents to an amazing degree. Helen Keller is one of the best examples. This heroic woman achieved impossible goals thanks to her incredible determination and tenacity. She did this mainly, or perhaps entirely, because forgetting herself, she wished to help others.

In addition to purely personal goals, you should make a point of having a part in important causes which benefit your fellow man and your community. The history of the world is the story of the struggle between good and evil, between generosity and selfishness. Identify your hopes and efforts with the cause of good. You are sure to be on the winning side, as good always wins in the end.

Merely reading this brief comment on the importance of positive thinking is hardly likely to produce a lasting effect on your attitude towards life and its problems. You should make a habit of reading books on developing positive attitudes and building spiritual strength. By far the best of these books is, of course, the Bible. Reading this wonderful book regularly cannot fail to give you confidence in the future and new strength to face your difficulties. The Bible is God's love letter to his children. He tells us of His love for us and His readiness to forgive all those who ask Him, no matter how serious their transgressions may be. He invites us to turn our lives over to His care and humbly ask Him to remove our shortcomings.

Do not become depressed over the setbacks in your life. Depression is a purely selfish emotion. Brooding over lack of money, health or other misfortunes serves no positive purpose The smallest act of kindness is worth more than all the money in the world. The Good Book says, "If you do nothing more than give a drink of water to someone in need you will not miss your reward." Your money and other possessions you cannot take with you, but you will be carried to heaven on the hands of those you have helped in this life. Christ said, "I love generous souls which forgetting themselves wish well to others!" He never mentioned any reward for those who make a lot of money, or have a wonderful time or achieve great power.

9   **Summary**

We shall now briefly discuss and summarize the main causes of cancer suggested by holistic doctors in Europe.

Toxicity And Cancer

As can be seen from the material presented in this book, it is becoming increasingly clear that cancer is not a disease at all. Many leading European holistic doctors now believe that far from being a dangerous disease, cancer is actually a natural method the body uses throughout life to cleanse itself of unwanted poisons and the wastes which are a by-product of metabolism.

The majority of toxins are disposed of by way of the regular channels of elimination—the liver, lungs, kidneys and skin. But some cells become so impregnated with poisons that they can no longer recover. These are the 100,000 cells that as suggested by Sir MacFarlane Burnet, can become cancerous each day.

Under normal conditions these cells are destroyed and eliminated together with the poisons they carry. However, if the body is weak and subjected to an overload of toxins, these poisoned cells cannot be eliminated fast enough. They begin to accumulate and form so-called malignant tumors. This is what Michio Kushi means when he says that "cancer is the body's healthy attempt to isolate toxins."

If the body can be strengthened and detoxified sufficiently, the accumulations of poisoned cells (cancerous tumors) are no longer necessary and the body breaks them down and eliminates them. This is what organized medicine calls "spontaneous remission." Most people are fooled by these scientific sounding words and they admire their doctor for his education and knowledge. They do not understand that in plain English "spontaneous remission" simply means "we haven't a clue what happened and we have no idea why this patient recovered."

Since a healthful life-style (i.e. one which strengthens the immune system) and cleansing are so useful in helping cancer patients, books on natural healing methods are full of stories of people who recovered from cancer. Some of the most important of these books are "A Cancer Therapy, Results Of Fifty Cases," by Dr. Max Gerson, "The Cancer Prevention Diet," by Michio Kushi, "Dr. Kelley's Answer To Cancer," by Dr. William Kelley and "The Grape Cure," by Johanna Brandt. These authors tell the stories of numerous terminal cancer patients who recovered when medical treatment was finally stopped and these patients' poisoned bodies were detoxified with strict cleansing diets. After reading these books it is impossible to come to any other conclusion, if one has any common sense at all, but that cancer is nothing more than a symptom of excessive toxicity and a weakened immune system. Cancer is simply a sign that the body is too weak to cope with the toxins which are being unloaded upon it—in the form of junk foods, chemicals, drugs, stimulants and other poisons. Dr. Gerson's book, "A Cancer Therapy, Results Of Fifty

Cases," is the best documented and scientific of the above four books. In this book Dr. Greson, a medical doctor who was ostracized by his profession because he preferred to use natural methods rather than drugs, tells how he was able to cure even the most advanced cases of cancer by using a strict cleansing program and natural health promoting foods.

The unwillingness of medical doctors to adopt cleansing methods for the treatment of cancer is in part understandable. They point out that cleansing is far from being a panacea and even Dr. Gerson did not succeed every time. As a result, the medical profession continues to search for its own cures for cancer in the faint hope that, some day, a remedy—a drug, vaccine or some procedure which can be entirely controlled by doctors—will be found to solve the problem of this deadly disease. However, if it is true that cancer is nothing but a symptom of toxicity and a weakened immune system, it is hard to see how a medical cure for cancer can ever be found. All the medical treatments for cancer used in the past, and it is unlikely that treatments used in the future will be much different, had four things in common. They weakened the patient further, they caused him to become even more toxic, they ruined him financially and, as a result, they aggravated the condition of everyone they were used on. If anyone accidentally recovered following the medical treatments, this was not because of the treatments but in spite of them. Some people were endowed with such remarkable vitality that they not only overcame the cancer but they also managed to survive the invasive medical treatments. This is confirmed by statistics which show that cancer patients who receive no medical treatment fare much better, and live longer, than those who receive orthodox medical treatments. But, somehow, organized medicine has managed to shuffle these statistics around in such a way that it appears as if doctors know what they are doing and that they are winning the "war on cancer."

Now that we know more about the causes of toxicity, it is clear why cleansing was not always successful in treating cancer. Although the cleansing programs used by Dr. Gerson and other famous doctors often produced wonderful results, they were only a limited approach. Many important forms of toxicity, which cannot be removed with the regular methods of cleansing, were overlooked.

Perhaps the methods of cleansing now used by European doctors who use electro-diagnosis have given us the best proof that cancer is only a symptom of toxicity. These doctors have found that symptoms of cancer, providing the disease is detected in time, invariably begin to disappear once the patient's body has been cleansed of parasites, funguses, yeasts, bacterial or viral infections, toxic metals (especially dental restorations made of toxic materials), harmful chemicals and other pollutants.

European doctors believe that cadmium is the most carcinogenic substance of all. This is because they have found cancer patients with cadmium toxicity cannot be cured until all the cadmium has been removed from their tissues. But once the cadmium has been removed, this can be easily accomplished with the help of homeopathic remedies, the cancer often regresses and disappears even if no treatment is used. On the other hand, even if a person shows the slightest signs of cadmium toxicity, beginning cancer can always be detected. Cadmium is found in paints, cosmetics, batteries and probably in many man-made chemicals.

Therefore, cadmium poisoning is not at all uncommon and it appears likely that this is the main reason for the tremendous increase in the incidence of cancer in modern times. Everybody would do well to have themselves checked regularly for cadmium toxicity. It has been suggested that if this were done the incidence of cancer could be cut by eighty to ninety percent.

As for the conventional methods for treating cancer which are used by organized medicine, they can best be described by using the old adage "the cure is worse than the disease." Invasive, senseless, barbaric medical intervention is often "the last straw that breaks the camel's back." In many cases, medical treatments for cancer leave a person in such an appalling condition that good health or permanent recovery are no longer possible. The deaths of many cancer patients are substantially hastened by the medical treatments they receive.

The medical treatments for cancer are so tragically unsuccessful because medical diagnostic methods are often unreliable. Lab tests, C.T. scans, M.R.I's and other diagnostic procedures used by doctors can be so inaccurate that they cannot pick up what is wrong until the problem has become catastrophic. If you doubt this statement, you should read the book "Confessions of a Medical Heretic," by Dr. Robert S. Mendelsohn, M.D., a leading physician who entitles his first chapter "Non Credo, (I do not believe in modern medicine!)" For instance, from this book you can learn, "right from the horse's mouth," about the doubtful value of lab tests. Dr. Mendelsohn writes, "to get some idea of what people are really getting for their $12 billion worth of lab tests each year, thirty-one percent of a group of laboratories tested by the CDC could not identify sickle-cell anemia. From ten to twenty percent of the tested groups incorrectly identified specimens as indicating leukemia...my favorite study is one in which a hundred and ninety-seven out of two hundred people were 'cured' of their abnormalities simply by repeating their lab tests."

What is perhaps even more important is that medical diagnostic methods give no clues as to the causes of cancer. As a result, they make it impossible to do anything about trying to prevent this dreadful disease. Because of this, medical treatments for cancer are only symptom-oriented. Not understanding what they are doing, medical doctors imagine that they are curing cancer when they destroy tumors. It never occurs to them that these tumors are far from being the real problem.

If it were not for electro-diagnosis and muscle-testing, a solution to the cancer problem may never have been found. These two methods have finally given us a clear understanding of the exact nature of cancer and of its underlying causes. As a result, cancer has now become one of the easiest conditions to prevent and nobody should have to die of this horrible disease anymore. Electro-diagnosis and muscle-testing make it possible to detect the disease

the moment it begins. In its early stages, cancer is very easy to cure and immediate action can be taken to get rid of it.

No progress can ever be made in the war against cancer until all doctors learn how to use electro-diagnosis or at least muscle-testing. Once these methods of diagnosis become accepted and widely used, cancer will be a thing of the past. The word CANCER will no longer strike terror in people's hearts.

Often the greatest problem facing the cancer patient is the cost of having his amalgam fillings and other toxic dental restorations replaced. The other healing professions are causing plenty of problems, but the prize has to go to the dentists. There can no longer be any doubt but that the toxic materials dentists place in patients' mouths kill more people and cause more trouble than what is being done by all the other healing professionals put together. Let us hope that dentists will finally become aware of the harm they are doing and that they will learn how to check whether the materials they are using are harmful to their unsuspecting patients. It is also about time dentists learn that with the adjustment of the atlas vertebra and good nutrition most cavities can be easily prevented.

Cancer And Yeast

There are two reasons why some researchers believe that cancer is nothing but a yeast, mold or fungus. Firstly, thanks to the work of such scientists as Dr. Paul Seeger, M.D., chemist, microbiologist and a candidate for the Nobel Prize, who found that the origin of cancer is often linked to the pathogenic forms of Mucor Racemosus Fresen and other fungi. Secondly, because it has been known for some time that in many cases tumors disappear rapidly when patients are given homeopathic remedies which <u>kill fungi, molds and yeasts</u>.

It is now known that these microorganisms are a normal part of the intestinal flora. They are always present in the body, and as long as we are in good health, and our immune system is strong, the body has little difficulty preventing them from spreading to areas where they do not belong. They only get out of control and begin to form tumors in persons who are weak and whose immune system is run down.

When it was first noticed that tumors often disintegrate and disappear if homeopathic remedies which kill yeasts, molds and fungi are used, some European holistic doctors began using these remedies routinely on their cancer patients. However, long term results were not encouraging. Although tumors shrank in many cases, they frequently grew back when the treatment was discontinued.

Consistently good results only began to be obtained when it was understood what causes yeasts, molds and fungi to invade parts of the body where they are not normally found.

It appears that the function of these microorganisms is to act as scavengers and help clean up and remove toxic wastes. If the body becomes excessively polluted, toxins begin to collect and eventually, if this situation is allowed to continue long enough, yeasts, fungi and molds may begin to grow on the accumulated waste. This may occur in one location or in several locations, either at the same time or at different times. (The advocates of this theory believe that this phenomenon has given rise to the belief that cancer is capable of metastases.)

Therefore, the first step in correcting the situation has to be a thorough cleansing of the body of all pollutants and poisons—i.e. parasites, bacteria and viruses, chemicals, toxic dental restorations, etc. By far the most important of these seems to be cadmium. For some reason as long as even the slightest traces of cadmium are present in a person's tissues it is impossible to kill yeasts, fungi and molds. Somehow, cadmium suppresses the body's ability to destroy these microorganisms and tumors will not go away.

This is what a European holistic doctor had to say about cadmium toxicity, "If it were not for the discovery of electro-diagnosis we would perhaps never have known how dangerous cadmium really is. Electro-diagnosis is such a sensitive diagnostic tool that, if used by an experienced doctor, it can detect cancer the moment the disease starts. For instance, in an experiment, some toothpaste, which was known to contain cadmium, was spread on a subject's hand. When this was done the beginnings of cancer could immediately be detected in the subject's body when he was checked with electro-diagnosis. All the signs of cancer disappeared again when the toothpaste was removed.

It is from experiments like this that we know that the presence of cadmium in the body somehow makes it impossible for us to fight cancer. If the cadmium is not removed cancer cannot be cured. On the other hand, if the cadmium is removed, this can best be done by using homeopathic remedies made specifically for this purpose, the cancer will often disappear even if no treatment for cancer is used.

There can be no doubt but that cadmium toxicity is the reason for the tremendous increase in cancer in our modern world. I have found cadmium in soaps, toothpastes, cosmetics, breath sprays, food preservatives, over the counter pain killing drugs, paints and even in the plastic that dentures are made of. Because cadmium is found in so many household items we are in constant danger of contamination. In two cases, I even found cadmium in the tap water patients were drinking. We just could not get them free of cadmium until they stopped using their tap water. Since then I always ask my patients to bring some of their water in gallon bottles for testing. In one such case I found no cadmium in the tap water but traces of it in water which had passed through a reverse osmosis water filter the patient had recently installed. As a result, I have had patients who were found to have cadmium poisoning many times in the course of a single year. You can remove it from their bodies with homeopathic remedies, but they soon pick it up again. When I see how many different commonly used items contain cadmium, I sometimes think there must be a conspiracy to put an end to the human race. Cancer is on the increase, soon over fifty percent of deaths will be caused by it."

The Immune System And Cancer

As we have already seen, the immune system plays an important part in defending us from cancer. Probably the most significant discovery made concerning the relationship of the immune system to cancer was that made by Sir MacFarlane Burnet in England. This outstanding Nobel Prize winning scientist found that about a hundred thousand cells become cancerous in the body every day of our lives. But if the immune system is strong and healthy it effectively destroys these cancerous cells so they cannot accumulate and form tumors.

Advocates of the theory that cancer is nothing but a symptom of a weak immune system argue that THIS CAN ONLY MEAN OUR IMMUNE SYSTEM CURES US OF CANCER EVERY DAY OF OUR LIVES. In other words, as long as we are in good health and our immune system is functioning normally—we can forget about cancer. When we are in good health our body is capable of easily dealing with cancer, without any outside help, and the disease can never develop and become life threatening. CANCER CAN ONLY DEVELOP IF THE BODY IS RUNDOWN AND THE IMMUNE SYSTEM WEAK.

From this we can see that, when treating cancer, it is not necessary to try to remove or destroy tumors. The body can do this easily without any help from doctors or anyone else.

The work of Dr. Lawrence Burton, and the immuno-augmentative therapy (IAT) which he developed after many years of research with a team of doctors and scientists in

New York, is perhaps the best proof of the tremendously important part the immune system plays in fighting cancer. When treated with IAT many of doctor Burton's patients recover even though the majority of them had been given up as terminal and untreatable by orthodox medicine. Many arrive at Dr. Burton's clinic in the Bahamas in such terrible condition they no longer have the strength to walk. They have to be carried in on stretchers. Yet they often recover when their immune system is strengthened with IAT. One of Dr. Burton's patients said, "a case that especially impressed me was that of a man with a large malignant tumor of the left lower lobe of the lung. After a few months of IAT this disappeared and his chest X-rays were clear. Another case with massive abdominal distention from ascites in a seemingly moribund and terminal condition also recovered and to all appearances seems cured. I have never seen anything like this occur with conventional therapies."

Dr. Burton uses specially prepared serums to strengthen his patients' immune system, but even a healthy, wholesome diet can be effective in boosting the immune system. This is why so many cancer patients have recovered when they were placed on a diet consisting almost entirely of raw vegetables, fruits and fruit juices. Vitamins and other nutritional supplements can also be helpful in strengthening the immune system and have also been used successfully in holistic cancer therapies.

However, this approach—i.e. different therapies to strengthen the immune system—was also frequently unsuccessful until it was understood that chemicals and parasites (worms, bacteria, viruses) can significantly inhibit a person's immune system. By far the most important is, of course, our old friend cadmium. At least as far as cancer is concerned, the presence of even the smallest traces of this metal in a patient's tissues make it impossible to cure him of this deadly disease. However, traces of nickel, lead, aluminum, pesticides, insecticides and other chemicals also help to weaken the immune system. If they can be removed with homeopathic remedies the probability of recovery has to increase.

When discussing this subject, it is impossible not to mention the effect of exercise on the immune system. It has been known for a long time that exercise, especially vigorous exercise, boosts the immune system enormously. In fact, recently the Federal government conducted a study of a large number of people over a period of several years to determine the relationship of exercise to the incidence of cancer and other degenerative diseases. Some startling discoveries were made. Amazingly, it was found that the incidence of cancer among women who did a lot of vigorous exercise on a daily basis was much lower than among women who exercised little.

This proves once again that cancer is not a disease in its own right, but only a symptom of a weak immune system. The lesson that can be learned from this is that if you WANT TO STAY ALIVE YOU MUST TRY TO STAY FIT AND IN GOOD PHYSICAL CONDITION.

Metals And Cancer

The last of these theories maintains that metals are the main cause of cancer. This is simply because cancer disappears so often after the removal of all metals—watches, jewelry (rings, bracelets, necklaces, etc.), dental restorations made of metals (amalgam fillings, gold crowns and inlays, etc.), metals in clothing (buckles, clasps, zippers, etc.) and especially traces of metals found in a person's tissues (lead, nickel, aluminum, cadmium, etc.). It appears that <u>metals disrupt normal body function more than</u> anything else.

Apart from cancer many other conditions usually improve or cease entirely when all metals are removed from patient's bodies—backaches, headaches, stiffness, knee pain, carpal tunnel syndrome, indigestion and even, this will surprise you, vitamin and mineral deficiencies.

With the knowledge that we now have, cancer has indeed become one of the most treatable and preventable conditions. When these new discoveries become widely used we will at last see THE END OF CANCER. However, this will not happen unless electro-diagnosis and muscle-testing are recognized as reliable methods of diagnosis and become widely used. Orthodox diagnostic methods are not sensitive or accurate enough, they often do more to mislead the doctor than to help him.

Prevention Of Cancer

With the knowledge that we now have cancer is very easy to prevent. European holistic doctors believe that it is virtually impossible to develop cancer if one does not have one or more of the following problems: amalgam fillings or any other toxic dental restorations, yeast, chemical poisoning, intestinal parasites, viral or bacterial infections or, most important of all, cadmium contamination.

Anyone interested in cancer prevention should be checked for these problems at least once every three months, either with electro-diagnosis or with muscle-testing. This only takes a few minutes but might save you endless problems.

The Soft Laser

Laser therapy, when used for healing, refers to the use of low level energy or "cold" laser to help promote tissue repair. Most of us, however, are more familiar with high-energy laser used for cutting metal or surgery. This is the so-called "hot" laser. Low-level laser, by contrast, will not heat up tissue. This is why it is called the cold laser. Instead, the tissues take in the laser energy and use it to speed up the healing process. Studies have shown that the cells in tendons, muscles and ligaments repair from 50 to 60 percent faster when laser therapy is used.

Laser energy increases circulation by dilating blood vessels and increasing the diameter of lymphatic ducts. It also has a significant effect on nerve cells by reducing the sensitivity of nerve endings and increasing the level of endorphins, the body's own pain blockers. As a result, areas of damaged tissues are not as sensitive or sore.

Injuries that involve sprains, strains or inflammation of muscle, tendon or ligament may be helped with laser therapy. Laser energy has also been shown to greatly reduce healing time in large skin wounds and to reduce the formation of scar tissue.

Recently it has been suggested by experts in Europe that the soft laser could play an important part in cancer prevention. This is because electro-diagnosis and muscle-testing have shown that the soft laser is capable of killing many parasites, bacteria and viruses as well as removing cadmium, nickel, mercury and many other toxic materials from body tissues. Since the above factors are the main causes of cancer in most people, it seems likely that regular use of the soft laser could play an important part in cancer prevention.

If you would like to know more about how muscle-testing can be used, you may be interested in Dr. Lubecki's book, *Now You Can Be Your Own Best Doctor.* This book explains simple methods of muscle-testing which can easily be learned by laymen.

You may also be interested in Dr. Lubecki's latest book, *There is a Cure for C.F.S.* (Chronic Fatigue Syndrome). This book explains how electro-diagnosis and muscle-testing have made it possible to discover the reasons for CFS and how this condition can be corrected. These books can be obtained from:

ProMotion Publishing
3368 F Governor Drive, Suite 144
San Diego, CA 92122